ECONOMIC SCARCITY AND HEALTHCARE QUALITY

Economic Scarcity and Healthcare Quality

Tradeoffs in Delineations and Dilemmas

LES SEPLAKI, Ph.D.

Dartmouth

Aldershot • Brookfield USA • Singapore • Sydney

Published by
Dartmouth Publishing Company Limited
Gower House
Croft Road
Aldershot
Hants GU11 3HR
England

Dartmouth Publishing Company
Old Post Road
Brookfield
Vermont 05036
USA

British Library Cataloguing in Publication Data
Seplaki, Les
 Economic scarcity and healthcare quality : tradeoffs in
 delineations and dilemmas
 1.Health care rationing
 I.Title
 338.4'3'3621

Library of Congress Cataloging-in-Publication Data
Seplaki, Les
  Economic scarcity and healthcare quality / Les Seplaki.
   p.   cm.
  Includes index.
  ISBN 1-85521-841-0 (hc)
  1. Medical economics. 2. Medical care.
 RA410.5.S366   1996
 338.4'33621--dc20   96-44639
                                                                          CIP

ISBN 1 85521 841 0

Printed in Great Britain by
Antony Rowe Ltd, Chippenham, Wiltshire

Contents

List of Abbreviations

AMA - American Medical Association

BC/BS - Blue Cross Blue Shield

CBA - Cost-Benefit Analysis

CEA - Cost Effectiveness Analysis

CON - Certificate of Need

CPI - Consumer Price Index

DRG - Diagnostic Related Group

EPO - Exclusive Provider Organization

ERISA - Employee Retirement and Income Security Act

FDA - Food and Drug Administration

FFS - Fee-for-Service

FTE - Full-time Equivalent

HCGA - Health Care Financing Administration

HMO - Health Maintenance Organization

IPA - Independent Practice Association

JCAHO - Joint Commission on Accreditation of Healthcare Organizations

LTC - Long-term Care

MCO - Managed Care Organization

NHI - National Health Insurance

NHS - National Health System

P.L. - Public Law

PPRC - Physician Payment Review Commission

PPO - Preferred Provider Organization

PPS - Prospective Payment System

RVS - Relative Value Scales

UCR - Usual, Customary and Reasonable

Preface

Healthcare quality is a highly subjective term which has different meanings for different people, depending upon the role and functions of those under consideration. Once it is defined, it needs to be measured so as to ascertain that members of society are receiving care of some prescribed quality or at least at some minimum standard. Yet, healthcare is an economic good. It is relatively scare. It is expensive, and has become increasingly so over the years. Traditionally, and to a large extent even today, medical care quality was often assessed in terms of the volume of care that was delivered. Even today, we note that different volumes of care may be delivered to different patients with apparently the same needs only because they have differing levels of financial resources. That may mean that different people are accorded differing care qualities both in terms of quantity and intensity of care. Major social and political issues arise. Healthcare, just like any other service or commodity, is produced at a cost. Larger delivered volumes of care normally generate higher costs, even at constant levels of technology. Increased technological applications will increase care costs even at the same quantity level. When both the quantity of delivered healthcare and the applied levels of technology increase, as they did in recent decades, healthcare costs spiral. Continuously spiraling healthcare costs bound to invoke socioeconomic and political concerns. Society is entitled to care at some level of quality. Furthermore, it is thought by many that all members of society are entitled to some level of care quality. However, given the cost of care, how should the scarce medical resources be distributed among members of society. To each according to his or her means? That would likely mean that care would be distributed according to wealth - not necessarily meaning that so would health and well-being, but that is another issue. Under this scenario, those with no means, the very poor and the indigent, could purchase none of this essential economic good called healthcare. However, most modern societies seem to advocate the entitlement to healthcare, some healthcare, by everyone. Once again, economics enters into the picture. How can scarce resources be stretched to cover everyone's needs? To answer that question, however, we need to know how "needs" should be defined, and then the "need" for what amount of healthcare, at what level of intensity. Given the scarcity of resources that society can allocate to medicine without seriously short-changing other economic and social endeavors, issues and serious reasoning pertaining to care quality under perennial cost-containment efforts tend to be circular and indefinite. Either the purse has to be larger, but not "too large", or the care has to be restricted, rationed or otherwise controlled - all subject to some standards of quality for all members of society. These are issues that clearly have the potential for outlasting both the providers and the recipients of healthcare on the one hand, and politicians as well as policy makers on other.

Chapter 1, **Introduction and Overview,** introduces the major issues in a broad setting. Concepts of healthcare quality in traditional and more modern contexts are introduced. Chapter 2, **Generic Notions of Product and Quality,** looks at how quality in general has been viewed in the literature, what the basic elements product quality are, and how product quality has been viewed and implemented in post-World War II industrial societies. Chapter 3, **Definitions and Delineations of Healthcare Quality**, examines in detail the issues and problems involved in identifying the concept and measuring healthcare quality. It also applies the basic theory of rational economic behavior to service choices in some healthcare endeavors, and looks at the social and policy implications of healthcare quality research. Of the various approaches to healthcare quality definitions, the one advanced by the National Academy of Sciences, Institute of Medicine, is concentrated upon. Chapter 4, **Measuring Healthcare Quality: Broad Issues**, presents an overview of some of the more prominent methods that research advanced in order to measure healthcare quality. In this connection the utility of regulatory efforts, relevant databases, and various quality indexes are looked at. In Chapter 5, **Measuring Healthcare Quality: Empiricisms**, various statistical techniques, specific health databases, and the empirical dimensions of outcome research are examined. Insurance claim files and the results of consumer surveys and patient feedbacks are also examined as vehicles for care quality measurement. Chapter 6, **Institutional Healthcare Quality**, looks at healthcare quality monitoring in hospital and other institutional healthcare environments. In particular, mortality rates as a yardstick for hospital care quality, and the impact of the Prospective Payment System are studied. The Chapter also examines healthcare quality at non-hospital institutional providers, and managed care entities. Chapter 7, **Healthcare Quality and The Individual Provider**, looks at quality issues in the physician's office, and the institutional as well as financial determinants of care supplied by private physicians. The chapter contrasts traditional fee-for-service environments with more contemporary capitation-based reimbursement arrangements with private and government payers, including the physician payment reforms, recently implemented by Medicare. The various HCFA maintained datafiles are briefly surveyed in terms of their possible contributions to healthcare quality assessment efforts. The relationships between the size of physician practice and care quality is also scrutinized. Chapter 8, **Cost–Quality Relationships**, examines the dichotomy between quality improvements and their consequences in terms of costs, and looks at the relationships between care quality and cost-benefit/cost-effectiveness analyses.

Chapter 9, **Monitoring Healthcare Quality by Assurance**, looks at the various principles and practices of quality insurance programs at hospitals. Inpatient mortality and care-based quality assurance models are looked at, and quality assurance projects both within and outside HCFA are examined. Chapter 10, **Monitoring Care Quality by Peer Review**, examines the functions of professional peer reviews in terms of assessing and improving care quality in private and public sector settings. The history and development of peer review efforts and their impact on quality are examined in hospital and other institutional healthcare, including managed care, settings. Chapter 11, **The Legal Environment for Healthcare: The Health-care Quality Improvement Act**, looks at the notions of needed and unneeded care in connection with care standard criteria. In particular, the ability of the courts to set care standards, and to measure deviations from those standards, are analyzed extensively within the context of contemporary medical malpractice litigation. The development and implementation of legislative remedies to blatant infringements on healthcare quality standards, particularly by way of the Health Care Quality Improvement Act, are analyzed. The Chapter also examines in depth the impact of the Act on the peer-review process, and the legal immunities accorded to peer-reviewers. HCQIA created the National Practitioners Data Bank. The Chapter also looks at the impact of the latter on physician practice quality. The last substantive chapter, Chapter 12, **The Legal Environment for Healthcare Quality: Competition Enforcement**, analyses in depth the impact of antitrust enforcement in the healthcare sector on healthcare quality, and the role of healthcare quality issues in antitrust litigation. The volume closes with a brief **Restatement and Conclusion** of the major issues, and with an important policy recommendation to the effect that managed care entities should be viewed as public utilities, and should be regulated as such.

The author benefited from interactions with a number of professionals and experts. H. McKillop, MD a Research and Clinical Fellow at the Mount Sinai Medical Center in New York was kind enough to share her thoughts with me on Chapters 3, 6 and 7. I thank C. Muller, Ph.D., also of Mount Sinai, for helpful comments on Chapters 5, 7, and 8. S. Ohm, MD of New York Down State Medical College, reviewed earlier versions of some of the material. M. Drach, Esquire, an attorney active in the New York medical malpractice litigation scene commented upon my analyses of related issues. Z. Marin, DDS., of NYU Dental School, shared her thoughts with me regarding various aspects of quality assurance, and peer review processes, in institutional settings. Last, but not least, D. Du, MD, Ph.D. was also kind enough to enlighten me by way of a number of conversations regarding some of the inner workings of institutional care quality control, quality assurance, and peer reviews. As a Visiting Scholar there while completing this volume, the author benefited substantially from the superbly organized and impressively endowed resources of the Columbia University Health Sciences Library in New York City. To announce the usual, that is, that all omissions, errors and other shortcomings of the volume remain the author's responsibility is virtually redundant.

1 Introduction and Overview

In the current system of US medical care delivery, with the threats or promises, depending on the eyes of the beholder, of healthcare reforms constantly in contention, cost containment has not only become but has long been a central issue. The implementation of cost containment efforts, in turn, has traditionally been envisioned either by way of enhanced competition in medical markets, or by intensified regulation, but was in fact seen in practice to emerge by way of the occurrence of both, increased competition *and* increased regulation[1]. In recent years, this dichotomy has been augmented by a third concern, healthcare quality, in the face of cost containment and regulation. The concern is that cost containment by way of increased competition and regulation on the healthcare scene is encouraged on the expense of healthcare quality. Thus, incentive programs implemented by proliferating HMOs link physician performance to service and technology utilization. The fixed patient fee based HMO capitation system discourages utilization so as to limit expenses (utilization) against revenues. Physician financial incentive systems reward those who underutilize and punish the overutilizers[2].

To cope with excessive utilization and resultant costs, third-party payers, state and federal governments, insurance companies and private employers implemented utilization review programs. These programs typically target hospital admissions, hospital inpatient-days, as well as hospital and total medical outlays. Traditionally, these programs have focused on the individual physician because historically individual physicians in private practice constituted the noninstitutional core of medical practice. Thus, programs were designed to seek out physicians who were under-trained, did not keep up-to-date hence were out-of-touch, abused substance, and demonstrated incompetence in a variety of other ways. In more recent times, these programs have lost relevance since the autonomy of the individual practitioner was shrinking and the institutional delivery of healthcare gained increased prominence[3]. Managed care of various forms have come to dominate the practice of medicine

Managed care institutions have historically "managed" care for the predominant purpose of controlling healthcare costs, with quality typically receiving secondary consideration. More recently, however, quality also began to receive some attention by providing quality-based incentives to physicians[4], and by research funding from federal and private organizations designed to establish complex databases for healthcare quality protection[5].

Healthcare Quality Views in Historical Contexts

As I suggested earlier, the historical burden of healthcare quality implementation has typically fallen on the individual practitioner, the doctor. Failure in proper implementation was thus attributed to the physician as an individual, and was analyzed in that context rather than institutionally. In fact, until a few years ago, malpractice cases were brought mostly against individual physicians and rarely against hospitals or other institutional providers[6]. Disciplinary actions by state licensing boards also concentrated mostly on the physician with staff privilege issues involving only private provider qualifications[7]. These can be viewed as pioneering efforts for quality assessment, although they were not adequate for measuring care quality system-wide. The problem rests with the notion that private physicians do not err often enough to produce a statistical base for classifying physicians into various quality of performance categories[8].

Additionally, arriving at an acceptable definition of "error" itself may be difficult. Traditionally, "error" meant deviation of some degree from accepted standard of medical practice within the community - which can be highly arbitrary and open to various interpretations, since accepted practice standards for any community are subjective notions. However, even if there were no measurement problems in this context, this view of performance may be seen as far too narrow for it does not explicitly include broader and just as important considerations such as historical patterns of private and community practice and outcomes, administrative procedures and frameworks for reviewing healthcare quality and performance, technological applications, practice styles, financial incentive systems [e.g. within HMOs] and resource constraints, as well as patient-physician relationships[9]. "Error" is also a relative term. It clearly indicates some action, or inaction, in relation to some standard for that action. Thus, some researchers define that *standard* in healthcare as an activity which at the least prevents a deterioration in health status and may even increase it in the face of a disease or condition[10]. Quality thus entails the proper selection of tasks or activities and their implementation with optimum outcome subject to constraints.

The setting is further complicated by the changed relationship between physicians and institutional providers. Traditionally, much of healthcare was delivered by hospitals either governed or owned by physicians. Recent trends changed much of this institutional setting to where physicians as well as hospitals and their staff function under the direction of outside institutional governing body that may not primarily be medical in nature although uses medicine for generating income and profits. Thus, hospitals and individual providers became employees, in a narrow but also frequently in a broad sense, of outside economic interests motivated primarily by profit constraints subjecting all of their other activities primarily to those constraints. Furthermore, as a source of even relatively major medical care service items, hospitals are often replaced by ambulatory free-standing care environments such as clinics, and emergy or surgi centers.

Although profit motive has gained momentum and continues its increasing domination of the healthcare environment, quality issues either for ethical or for legal reasons, or both, are also gaining prominence. *Quality assessment* and *quality assurance* are now heavily weighted factors in providing medical care both in private and institutional environments. Healthcare assessment ground work appears to have been implanted by way of three principles: structure, process and outcome[11]. *Structure* focuses on the physical environment and tools utilized in healthcare, such as personnel qualifications, administrative structures, and procedure implementation. *Process* is typically seen as patient specific treatment dimensions and the way medical personnel function in an institutional setting. Peer-based evaluations are normally performed in terms of some relative community based standards, although admittedly the latter themselves may not have been adequately assessed. Finally, there is thought to be a relationship between process and *outcome*, although the nature of that relationship is by no means defined. Outcome measurements are aimed at determining if the patient has become better, at least in his or her perception, and at the minimum at ascertaining that the patient has not become worse as a result of implemented healthcare procedures.

Assessing healthcare outcome entails considerable difficulties. Much of outcome assessment needs to isolate those factors and their impact which were involved in the care itself from those which are external to the care process. We can thus differentiate between endogenous healthcare factors and those that are exogenous. The task is to identify these factors, separate them, and assess their respective impact on the patient during and subsequent to the implementation of the care. There are significant time dimensions to account for as well. These parameters carry their inherent measurement problems as outcomes (except very explicit ones such as death) in general are difficult to measure. If death is not part of the outcome, then factors such as patient attitudes, state of post treatment psychology, post treatment social status, and the like, all need to be measured - a difficult task. Furthermore, even if measurability was a relatively easy task, the cost of data generation and aggregation maybe quite significant and case specific cost-benefit analyses may be warranted to perform such tasks. The problems in this context are further compounded by the likely need to take measurements at different times after the completion of the treatment process (provided such "completion" does occur), each time needing to incur the costs and needed cost-benefit analyses. Additionally, the results of one study at one time may impact upon or even cause continuing altering or re-implementing care thus impacting later outcome measurements. Finally, but clearly nonconclusively, even if these measurements are performed serious difficulties may be encountered in relating specific outcome elements to specific treatment elements and the direction of causal relationships among these or even among various outcome elements. These and similar dilemmas should help us set the stage for this volume. Clearly, we will raise many more questions than generate answers. However, society and its professionals cannot produce answers without generating questions. Hence, refer to the title of the volume. Institutionally, much of healthcare quality measurements are implement through HCFA generated hospital mortality and morbidity data. The Joint Commission on the Accreditation of Healthcare Organizations (JCAHO) in turn utilizes this data in its accreditation process[12].

I indicated that the traditional healthcare quality spotlight has focused mostly on the physician. There were various target areas usually seen as various forms of malpractice. The most flagrant one involved patient and substance abuse, and medical state licensing boards and procedures often sought out symptoms of such conduct[13]. In addition, the Health Care Quality Improvement Act (1986) mandated healthcare databank (to be examined extensively in the volume) is designed to disseminate conduct specific information nation-wide[14]. A lower ranked malfeaser is the provider who, due perhaps to heavy work schedules, other preoccupations, or to preferences for various leisure-based activities does not keep up with new developments in the field, hence deviates from generally accepted community practice standards. Another negative performance dimension is the frequency of errors committed by a physician usually identified by hospitals and outside reviewers using aggregated data. Negative outcome patterns often appear to concentrate on a small repeater group of practitioners[15].

Treatment process and outcome are also a function of statistical considerations on the part of the provider. There is variability in treatment outcomes. The patient's condition may deteriorate because he or she *was* treated in the same manner and to the same extent as if he or she was not treated. Similarly, the patient may experience improvement pursuant to treatment in the same manner as without treatment. Thus, when applying treatment, or otherwise, the physician is essentially playing some odds. The risk-outcome quality trade-off is constantly present, although to varying degrees depending on the patient's prevailing condition. A diagnosis places the patient into a class of a frequency distribution along with the relevant probabilities for treatment outcomes. The benefit is that the patient is no longer viewed as a random occurrence with his or her welfare depending on the physician's personal intuition. The downside, on the other hand, is inherent in the statistical uncertainties and probabilities involved with the outcome for a particular treatment[16].

Clinical decisions often carry a risk. The notion that a treatment cannot hurt may not be valid, as many treatments can hurt, drugs carry side effects, hospitalized patients are vulnerable to infections, and surgeries (particularly under general anesthesia) carry the risk of complications, disability and even death. Clinical decisions entail costs. Misdiagnosed ailments can generate pecuniary and nonpecuniary costs to the patient, institutional providers, the physician and to society. Notwithstanding professional self-regulation, medical licensing and quality control procedures designed to cope with flagrant abusers, there is still a general problem with quality. Even among physicians who are generally viewed as competent omissions by way of missed diagnoses, unmonitored or inadequately monitored treatments, and unnecessary procedures, are still too frequent[17]. Recently emerged competitive pressures and institutionally imposed controls, such as may be seen with increasing frequency at HMOs, can contribute remedies to this predicament, as we will note later.

Medical *practice style* variations is also a source of concern, for these must be viewed in the light of prevailing practice standards. Adequate information seems to be lacking regarding the nature, extent and causes for these variations and regarding their consequences for care quality. Nor there appears to be in place an adequate mechanism designed to secure the necessary flow of feedback to practitioners regarding the quality of their practice. Government efforts and resources may provide part of the answer.

The Medicare program provides considerable data regarding treatment outcomes. The recently established practitioners databank contains some information regarding the most prominent negative dimensions of past practice patterns. Finally, modern computer software is designed to maintain and track patient information[18].

Healthcare Quality in the Medical Industrial Society

Given the affiliation of most physicians with one or more institutions, and in many cases physicians being on full-time staff of institutions, the emerging dominance of group practices, PPOs, HMOs, and hospital chains, much of the quality improvement and maintenance burden falls on these institutions. Prevailing payment systems, such as Medicare's DRG and some HMO's financial incentive structure, have often been blamed for healthcare quality reductions, and we have already alluded to them. May there be a relationship between the institutional structure and quality of practice, although not necessarily independent from payment systems? It may be that institutional settings, pressures, policies and politics play an important ultimate role in healthcare quality[19].

Many of these institutional settings rest upon indeed motivated by financial incentives for profits, hence controlling costs. Sophisticated computers and other tracking systems monitor physician practice, in particular diagnostic test patterns. An underlying assumption in the design of these monitoring systems is that human beings respond to financial incentives, placing physicians in a conflict situation: their own financial interest (closely tied to the financial interest of their employing institution) and the welfare of their patients. Further, it is not so much a specific institutional structure or legal form that impacts upon healthcare quality as the financial incentives which the institutions weave into their relationships with physicians. It may be that if these financial incentives drove some practitioners to compromise quality, then peer pressure (review procedures) often found in group practice, hospital and managed care environments will counteract that tendency to compromise quality for financial incentives[20]. In addition, even if they are not formally trained in medicine, institutional administrators, may go a long way by way of intense review procedures in imposing quality controls on practitioners. We will not at this time discuss the downside of strict administrative controls by way of negative physician reactions and compromised practitioner morale. Nonetheless, some or even extensive loss of professional autonomy on the part of physicians may be a small price to pay if enhanced administrative controls yield long-run benefits to the patients and to the physician's employer.

The cause is further enhanced by active physician participation and involvement in the administrative decision-making process itself. Studies have shown a positive relationship between the extent to which physicians have actually been involved in an institution's decision-making process and the quality of care delivered subject to imposed cost constraints[21]. Furthermore, recent approaches employed by managed care organizations (HMOs, PPOs, etc.) tended to focus on *outcomes management* (quality assessment and feedback), well beyond traditional cost controls. Outcome management is implemented by integrating the forces relevant to assessing healthcare quality. This integration may be embodied in a permanent national medical database utilizing a common set of definitions for measuring the quality of care and the quality of life. The national database would utilize a language easily understood by laymen as well as medical professionals, and would contain information on health outcomes, as well as related financial and administrative dimensions. It would present a readily understandable picture of the relationship between treatment, health outcome, and related financial consequences, all viewed within the context of some standards for the relevant medical practice[22]. These issues will be dissected in the following chapters of this volume.

What is Healthcare Quality After All?

Defining and measuring healthcare quality is often an elusive task. But one wonders why we should be concerned with healthcare quality as the US enjoys probably the most sophisticated and highest quality of medical care, stated in broad terms, throughout the world. Our physicians are generally well trained both in academic and clinical environments. In addition, as I noted earlier, there are some safeguards built into the medical care delivery system designed to check quality. In spite of this favorable appearance, there are many pitfalls and problems with the quality of healthcare delivery. While these problems may not be apparent to most of the "average" patients, in fact most patients by themselves would be incapable of discerning quality problems, these problems become evident from specialized studies and the review of the literature. It also becomes evident from the high frequency of medical malpractice law suits. Although apparently some two-thirds of these suits are lost by the complainants, many are won, huge verdicts are brought by the courts attempting to compensate the victim and rewarding a relatively few members of the judiciary. In addition, still rapidly increasing healthcare expenditures, consequent cost-containment efforts and closely managed service utilization generate further concerns and questions regarding the current status and future fate of quality on health services delivery. More on that later.

The delivery of healthcare services and scrutinizing the results of that delivery is a complicated process even in a simple fee-for-service doctor-to-patient direct relationship. Thus, when one attempts to discern what the outcome(s) of a treatment or a series of treatments happen(s) to be, the researcher is faced with a web of complex scientifically interrelated, but often unknown or even unpredictable labyrinth of cause-effect relationships, sometimes unilateral but often running in bilateral and even multilateral directions, compounded and further complicated by the third dimension of time and timing, both as to treatment(s) and to outcome(s). If this was not complex enough, in most treatment processes and outcomes elements of personal and human relationships enter, the patient's perception of the physician and vice versa, as well as the patient's perception of the treatment which can impact, albeit quite immeasurably, both on the treatment and on the outcome of the treatment. Accepting the frequently quoted assertion that "medicine is as much of an art as a science" implants additional fear and uncertainty in the mind and heart of researchers who attempt to define and quantify healthcare quality. The scrutiny of the "art" aspect of the definition may rest on the psychological rapport, i.e. trust, between the physician and the patient, with the latter, in turn, depending on such dubiously measurable notions as compassion, respect and integrity - obviously perceptions in the eyes of the beholders. The emergence of large managed care organizations limiting the choice of physicians thereby imposing impersonal, efficiency hungry profit driven providers on their patients must clearly play havoc with the "art" component of care quality definitions. While traditionally patients were to see their physicians as their agents and advocates, managed care environments at least in their traditional form raised questions as to the physicians' primary interest and concern being their own financial and those of the managed care organization, with patient's welfare coming a distant third.

In order to render the task of healthcare quality definition and measurement somewhat manageable, we will find in this volume that most studies see the process as a simple relationship between the cause: the treatment, and the effect: the outcome. It is further assumed that if the former is properly applied the latter will be optimum, although in recent years this "optimum" has been subjected to resource constraints. The quality of care is simply judged in terms of the quality of the result. While earlier efforts saw quality within the context of the technical delivery of care only, more recent assessments include consumer reactions[23]. Furthermore, with the institutionalization of medical care delivery where physicians function within health systems and large managed care organizations, the clinical definition of the quality of care tends to expand to include not only the technical performance of the physicians but the overall performance of the entire healthcare delivery system as well.

Within an institutional environment physician performance can readily be assessed, even continuously audited, by the application of a *treatment protocol system (tps),* particularly in situations involving difficult treatment and ethical issues. TPS has long been used by nurses and other healthcare providers whose function is largely subject to physician supervision. It is a set of predetermined flow-chart based instructions covering the care management of a patient with a specific problem. Given the patient's symptoms and signs, the healthcare worker is essentially taken by the hand by the computer program containing the TPS (sometimes also called "clinical algorithms") and dictates at each step of the way what the next action should be, where findings at each step contribute to the determination of what the next step should be. These TPSs may now be used for guiding and simultaneously auditing physician diagnostic and treatment performance in relation to some generally accepted standards of care[24], and may contribute to a reduction in practice style variations. Indeed, some studies have found an almost automatic improvement in the statistical quality of diagnosis and care by using computerized sophisticated treatment protocols which proved themselves to be more reliable than private physicians professional but discretionary decisions[25].

Healthcare Quality and Some Legal Issues

The concern for quality of care practiced by the private physician has been extended throughout the institutional and corporate environment of the practitioner. Thus, institutions have been held liable for the omissions or commissions of private doctors functioning within their confines. Physicians have typically not been viewed by the courts as independent contractors. Institutionalized medicine's heavy regulation and the need for supervision over physician activities were viewed as dominant. Thus, a court imposed liability on the entire hospital for the malfeasance of its emergency room physician, although the latter was an independent contractor[26]. The hospital was seen as the bearer of ultimate responsibility for what transpires within its institutional confines, and the court compared the hospital's responsibility to that of a common carrier to protect its passengers. In another case of the same year, a similar liability theory was extended to HMOs[27], and a court on appeal rejected the institution's argument that its physicians practiced independent medicine and that it could not control their diagnostic judgments and treatment decisions. A third decision applied the doctrine of corporate negligence when the injury was sustained by the patients from physicians who were not hospital employees[28]. If the hospital has actual knowledge of the procedures performed within its institutional confines it is normally held liable for a negative outcome. It appears in general that as the sophistication and coverage of medical practice databases broadens, so does the hospital's responsibility to avoid competence and performance gaps in its staff.

An often used legal aspect of practicing medicine is *informed consent*: disclosure of diagnosis, the nature of treatment and the risks involved. It is essentially designed to foster patient-doctor relationship and to protect the provider against claims that risks of negative results were not disclosed, hence the patient was not in the position to make informed decision. It was argued, however, that in spite of informed consent disclosures, the patient may not become aware of all the important information in a timely fashion, nor does he or she understand or even become intelligently cognizant of all of the risks involved[29].

In New York State, *mandated recredentialing* to deal with practitioners whose original training has been rendered obsolete due to advances in their fields with which they have not kept up received considerable attention[30]. Mandated recredentialing of physicians active in delivering healthcare is considered necessary every nine years, although thus far no strong link has been established between the practice and marked improvement in care quality. On the other hand, the relevance of the science of medicine, if not the art of it, does depreciate quite rapidly pursuant to new studies and discoveries not only of new diagnostic and treatment processes but also of the harmful effects of old ones. In view this trend, mandated recredentialing will likely increase quality standards in medicine.

Managed Care and Care Quality

Given the legal liability of managed care organizations for the practice of their affiliated providers, and notwithstanding the frequently held traditional view of HMOs as sources of relatively poor care, quality issues particularly in terms of outcomes for HMOs and their actual as well as potential customers have come to the foreground. Indeed, under these emerging circumstances, HMOs may be seen not as sources of relatively poor care or poor outcome but rather those with a better potential for care quality improvements.

Care quality can be a potent marketing tool, designed to attract those many additional customers ("members") which HMOs need in order to succeed in a competitive healthcare delivery environment. The very nature of many HMOs' policy of not securing provider choice for their members will likely generate the necessary uncertainty on the part patients not present with established choice providers that will prompt them to investigate an unknown physician's competence. To accommodate actual and potential customer inquiries, HMOs may generate performance and outcome databases regarding their affiliated providers, if they have the resources to do so. Thus, while the HMO may put internal utilization constraints on its physicians in order to prompt them to keep costs down, they can induce and educate their consumers to place an external quality constraint upon the same physicians to keep quality up even in the face of utilization constraints. If this pair of endogenous/exogenous constraints, which we may label as the *"efficiency-quality dichotomy"*, is properly balanced and effectively administered, HMOs may indeed become a major source of healthcare quality improvement rather than sources of quality deterioration. Much will be said about this later in the volume.

This favorable outcome may be compounded by the availability of government generated outcome data for hospitals which enhances the HMO's ability to chose among institutional providers. Given the publicity periodically given to hospital mortality and morbidity statistics, the choice of institutional providers by an HMO becomes an integral part of its marketing policy as well as a predictor of its financial success. Thus, outcome related data and information for managed care systems and hospitals are becoming increasingly public domain. Federal, state and local governments become aware of them and respond to them through the market of public health patients. Employers become aware of them and respond through choice of outside providers (or lack thereof due to establishing their own clinics) as part their fringe-benefit package. And, with appropriate education and training and amply annotated dissemination techniques, patients become aware of them and respond by simple and traditional market choices.

The *efficiency-quality dichotomy* places physicians and institutional providers into a multidimensional state of responsibility where in order to remain a member of the team providers will have meet these responsibilities, particularly since functioning outside the managed care team is already becoming economically less feasible. An important additional aspect of the *efficiency-quality dichotomy* in managed care organizations is the application of a cluster of peer review processes where providers examine in an organized though competitive setting each other's performance and outcome in delivering medical services. Peer reviews may be implemented informally by an exchange of verbal notices, collegial pressures (even by withholding referrals) among physicians regarding their performance and errors. Or, as is often the case, it is implemented formally through organized, established and legally sanctioned and mandated procedures via the committee system. Thirdly, peer reviews may actually be imposed publicly upon assumed or actual negative performers through the medical malpractice litigation process whereby physicians express their professional opinion, usually for a fee, regarding various negative dimensions of another physician's performance.

"Peer review" by medical malpractice litigation is probably not the most efficient or even most effective method of attempting to measure or improve healthcare quality. First of all, the process is expensive from a social point of view; taxpayer funds are tied up for weeks sometimes for months while conducting the trial itself in the court of law, with publicly employed judicial professionals and their support staff being involved full-time. This follows many months and even years of expensive discovery and legal maneuvers which follow the initial filing of the complaint, once again often tying up publicly financed professional and para-professional time, as well as generating substantial expenditures on the part of the participants. The opinions expressed at trial, usually for jury consumption, are paid for. Medical experts, on both sides of the litigation, opine for a fee. The testimonies are often convoluted, technically complex, and probably confusing for juries which have to listen to them for days or weeks. The decision as to which medical expert's opinion ultimately prevails often depends not only (or perhaps not at all) on the purported competence of the medical experts, but on the impressions they leave with the jury, their personality, the personality and competence of the lawyers involved, the testimony and personality of other witnesses, and the general nontechnical impressions that the complainant(s) and the defendants generate with the jury. Poor medical performance may be upheld as correct, perfectly competent medical performance may go down on the records as having been incompetent and constituted malpractice, that is, if the court and the experts have succeeded in establishing the medical standards in relation to which the defendant's performance is usually adjudicated. If the litigated medical malpractice matter ends up not being tried for some reasons, the most common of which is settlement, then society's interests in uncovering and eliminating negative medical performances even by way of this imposed peer review process does not get served. Indeed, some settlements include formal, legally enforceable barriers to information dissemination regarding the defendant physician's performance that was the subject of the litigation in the first place.

While public disbursements on the case may turn out to be smaller, everyone benefits, except society. The attorneys get their fees, the expert services utilized get paid for, the claimant gets some money which amounts to more than if the case would have proceeded to a defense verdict, the defendant (or his or her insurance company) needs to disburse funds likely less than if the case would have proceeded to a plaintiff's verdict, everyone is satisfied to various degrees, but society's interests are largely dropped out of sight.

Under these circumstances, we do not find out if the quality of healthcare delivery was compromised, or even what the defendant physician actually did, and whether or not his or her performance was up to the parity dictated by accepted community practice standards. The physician returns to practicing medicine with the distinct possibility that if he or she malpracticed in the first instance that malpractice will likely be repeated again but at that time possibly without a recourse or without anyone taking any remedial action.

Thus, medical malpractice litigation, while potentially an effective policing weapon against gross malfeasers in the practice of medicine with its existence clearly justified by traditional failures within the medical profession to adequately police itself against its own members, may also be a source of substantial economic waste from society's point of view. While attorneys are entitled to reasonable fees, and a justified claimant winner is entitled to reasonable recovery, and the malpractitioner should be punished notwithstanding the financial shields afforded by the insurance carrier, the relevant medical malpractice judicial process should consider society's rather than private interests as paramount, and should contribute to the improvement in the quality of healthcare delivery instead reinforcing its status quo[31].

Peer reviews implemented in institutional settings appear to yield much better cost-benefit results for society. Some hospitals have a wide range of committees addressing performance issues such as morbidity, mortality, infections, pharmaceuticals, incident reports, utilization frequencies, and so forth. In addition, the JCAHO, Medicare under DRG, and other federally mandated PROs (professional review organizations) can all be utilized to affect physician performance reviews. Beyond its 1960 peer review mandate under the Medicare program by way of PROs, Congress has since mandated peer reviews in various managed care and competitive medical plans (CMP) settings. PROs under contract with the Federal Government evaluate provider utilization and quality serving the Medicare covered population, and their goals are enhanced by privately engaged review committees.

Intra-institutional quality oriented peer reviews are augmented by formal decisions regarding a practitioner's staff privileges. The latter may be denied on first application, revoked from continuation, or restricted by peer composed review committees thus implementing decisions aimed at care quality improvements. These reviews, in turn, are facilitated by The Health Care Quality Improvement Act of 1986 which mandated the establishment of a national computer databank (a registry) of practicing physicians, hospitals, and healthcare workers.

Before proceeding to the analyses of specific healthcare product quality definitions and measurements, I will next examine the generic notions of a "product" and "product quality" in some detail.

Notes

1. Seplaki, L., *Cost and Competition in American Medicine: Theory, Policy and Institutions*, University Press of America, Lanham, MD, 1994. See Ch. 28.
2. See for instance Knapp v. Palos Community Hospital 465 N.E.2d 554, 561 (Ill. App Ct 1984), where a staff physician's reappointment was denied by a hospital because the doctor was found to have used too much diagnostic tests, medications, and pulmonary angiograms, causing a 30% increase in costs.
3. Savard, P. and Gallagher, L., "Reflections on Change in Medical Practice: The Current Trend to Large Scale Medical Organizations", *JAMA,* Vol. 250, 1983, pp. 2820-2822.
4. Carlsen, B., "HMOs Try New Doctor Incentive: Quality Care Bonuses", *HealthWeek*, August 8, 1988, p. 22.
5. These databases will be examined later in the volume.
6. Furrow, B., Johnson, S., Jost, T. and Schwartz, R., *Health Law: Cases, Materials and Problems*, Foundation Press, New York, 1987.

7.   Kollmorgen v. State Board of Medical Examiners 416 N.W.2d 485-491 (Minn. App. 1987) involving overprescription of medicine.

8.   The volume will later examine an attempted solution for this dilemma by way of the Practitioners Databank.

9.   See for instance Wennberg, J., "Dealing with Medical Practice Variations: A Proposal for Action", *Health Affairs*, Vol. 3, No. 2, 1984.

10. Brook, J. and Kosecoff, K., "Commentary: Competition and Quality", *Health Affairs*, Vol. 7, No. 3, 1988.

11. Donabedian, A., "Evaluating the Quality of Medical Care", *Milbank Memorial Fund Quarterly*, Vol. 44, 1966. See also Donabedian, A., "Promoting Quality Through Evaluating the Process of Patient Care", *Medical Care*, Vol. 6, 1968.

12. We will take a closer look at the JCAHO. See also USGAO GAO/PEMD-88-23 1988, *Medicare: Improved Patient Outcome Analyses Could Enhance Quality Assessment*, and Office of Technology Assessment; US Congress, OTA-J-952 1988, *The Quality of Medical Care: Information for Consumers,*.

13. McAuliffe, J., Rohman, K. et al, "Psychoactive Drug Use Among Practicing Physicians and Medical Students", *New England Journal of Medicine*, Vol. 315, 1986, p. 805. See also Guinther, J., *The Malpractitioners*, Anchor Press, Garden City NJ, 1978.

14. Health Care Quality Improvement Act of 1986 42 U.S.C. 11101-35, (Supp. IV, 1986).

15. Brook, R., Williams, K., "Evaluation of the New Mexico Peer Review System: 1971-73", *Medical Care (Supp)*, Vol. 14, 1976.

16. Jennet, B., *High Technology Medicine: Benefits and Burdens*, Oxford University Press, New York, 1986. See also Jonsen, K., "Teaching the Ethics/Technology Interface", *International Journal of Technological Assessment*, Vol. 3, 1987; Eddy, L., Variations in Physician Practice: The Role of Uncertainty", *Health Affairs*, Vol. 3, 1984.

17. Lohr, K., *Quality of Care in Episodes of Common Respiratory Infections in A Disadvantaged Population*, Rand Paper Series #P6570, 1980.

18. Paul-Shaheen, K., Clark, J. and Williams, L., "Small Area Analysis: A Review and Analysis of the North American Literature", *Journal of Health Policy, Politics and Law*, Vol. 12, 1987.

19. Friedson, E., *Profession of Medicine: A Study of the Sociology of Applied Knowledge*, Harper & Row, New York, 1970.

20. A later chapter will be entirely devoted to the trade-off between cost control and care quality. See also Wolinsky, F. and Marder, W., *The Organization of Medical Practice and the Practice of Medicine*, Health Administration Press, Ann Arbor, MI, 1985.

21. Shortell, K., "Physician Involvement in Hospital Decision Making" in Gray, B. (ed), *The Health Care for Profit: Doctors and Hospitals in a Competitive Environment*, The National Academy Press, Washington, DC, 1983. Also see Neuhauser "Budgeting Incentives for the Appropriate Use of Medical Technology", *International Journal of Technological Assessment in Health Care*, Vol. 3, 1987.

22. These issues received pioneering treatment in Ellwod, "Shattuck Lecture - Outcomes Management: A Technology of Patient Experience", *New England Journal of Medicine*, Vol. 318, 1988.

23. See for instance HCFA's release of hospital specific mortality data which is often seen largely as a response to the "consumer's need to know". Also, the American Association of Retired Persons (AARP) prevailed upon the boards of Medicare peer review organization (PROs) to include patient group representatives; Lohr, K.N.,

"Commentary: Professional Peer Review in a 'Competitive' Market Model", *Case Western Reserve Law Review*, Vol. 36, 1985-86.

24. Margolis, K., "Uses of Clinical Algorithms", *JAMA*, Vol. 249, 1983.

25. Goldman, Cook, Brand (and 18 other authors) "A Computer Protocol to Predict Myocardial Infraction in Emergency Department Patients With Chest Pain", *New England Journal of Medicine*, Vol. 318, 1988.

26. Jackson v. Power 743 p.2d 1376 (Alaska, 1987).

27. Sloan v. Metropolitan Health Council of Indianapolis Inc. 516 N.E.2d 1104 (Ind. Ct. App. 1987).

28. Thompson v. Nason Hospital 370 Pa. Super 115, 535 A.2d 1177 (1988).

29. Katz, J., *The Silent World of Doctor and Patient*, Free Press, New York, 1984; see also Lidz, C., Meisel, A. et al, *Informed Consent: A Study of Decision Making in Psychiatry*, Guilford Press, New York, 1984.

30. New York State Department of Health, *Report of the New York State Advisory Committee on Physician Recredentialing, Phase One: General Principles, Proposed Process, Recommendations*, 1988.

31. I will spend considerable time on the economics and various other dimensions of medical malpractice litigation in the last two chapters of the volume.

2 Generic Notions of Product and Quality

The source of need for standardized measures for healthcare quality appears to have been the insurance industry where cost and to an extent quality monitoring has in some form or another been a part of sound business practice. Input classification systems, such as the Medicare DRGs which assume a given amount of resource utilization per ailment for each patient admitted into the hospital, also enabled administrators and third-party payers to profile clinical activities within the hospitals. On the other hand, patient treatment and health progress in alternative facilities such as doctor's offices, hospitals, rehabilitation centers, nursing homes and other similar environments was not considered particularly essential. This approach may have been patterned after often used European practices where each patient's case management entails so called "capitation quotes", that is, the amount of resources made available for each patient[1]. The hospital has been replaced by the community in terms of resource management and control and is no longer the scene for the treatment for complete disease cycles. In other words, the focus of complete patient treatment cycles was transferred from the hospital into an institutional *network* environment where the continuity of patient care throughout the care cycle and the integration of communication among the elements of the network (the various facilities, institutions, providers) came into prominence. Decision methods and so called matrix-based models have become necessary (originally developed for solving industrial problems) for focusing on the patient as an entity independent from the various institutional and healthcare facility stages that the patient may pass through[2].

In this healthcare network, quality and cost may be examined by looking at the effects of diagnostic and therapeutic medical care episodes on the patient's health status, taking also into consideration the patient's perceptions of these care episodes. Thus, in a Donabedian sense, care "outcome" may be seen as the actual and perceived effect of any single care episode, or that of a collection of care episodes, upon the patient's health status - however the latter may be perceived, measured or expressed[3]. However, the design of hundreds of clinical trials to assess the outcome of any medical decision by individual physicians or care facilities on a case-by-case basis is clearly not feasible. Matrix based input-output models may come to the rescue.

Inputs may be viewed as anything that is provided by the facility to produce its output. These include staff, professional and paraprofessional personnel, consumable and long-term durable items, in-house services, administrative factors, and the like utilized within the facility. Output, on the other hand, may constitute actions taken and products produced by the organization in relation to a patient in order to generate a positive expected or desired health status for that patient, or, which is essentially the same, in order to avoid or prevent a negative expected health status. An accurate process of measuring inputs, outputs, and outcome must assume an accurate identification of the *unit of measurement,* enabling cross-system comparisons and correct policy decisions with respect to resource allocation. Healthcare *quality* would be expressed in terms of or in relation to some community or compliance standards or similar universally accepted yardsticks of measurement, in terms of all three dimensions, input, output and outcome. In other words, quality standards are seen in terms of the extent to which the healthcare network and its participants have delivered the desired results, with the designated resources, in relation to expectations or targeted standards.

In addition to, or instead of the DRG system of care classification, medical activities maybe unitized based on the so called *profiles of care* models[4]. This is premised on the understanding that in general initial patient complaints and symptoms as presented to the physician or in the hospital emergency room may be the main determinants of costs and resource designation related to a specific case, and not discharge specific diagnoses. If so, predefined and designated blocks of symptoms, and/or intermediate diagnoses at the referring physician level, linked up with their related procedures and objectives, maybe the basis for some type of quality control. That control can be expressed in terms of the deviation between some predetermined standards or expected outcomes on the one hand and observed consequences, on the other. The same may also serve as a basis for resource allocation decisions, and possibly case-mix management. This approach further assumes that the traditional aversion of physicians to administrative interferences with their practice will be overcome to the extent that complete physician cooperation and participation in the implementation of these systems can be assumed. Let us now take a look at some of the issues related to generic "product" and "product quality" considerations.

The Product and Its Quality

Product quality in general commerce has traditionally been considered as an important competitive variable in the market place. In recent years, its importance has gained momentum in the delivery of medical services as well. Yet, the general literature reflects some lack of comprehensive reviews of the notions of quality in general and that in healthcare. Part of the reason perhaps rests with the diversity of intellectual interpretations that the notion of quality can be subjected to. Philosophers are interested in the concept probably mostly from the point of view of defining it. Economic scholars might see quality as something closely related to profit maximization in a competitive market place and ultimately within the context of general market equilibrium. People who work in the field of marketing, on the other hand, could see quality as an important determinant of consumer behavior in the market place both in a perceived and experienced sense. Nonetheless, issues such as determining whether "quality" is subjective or objective in nature, whether or not it is socially determined and if so directly or indirectly, what its determinant and determined variables are, may overlap all disciplines. In economics the primary concern is obviously with relationships such as those between quality and cost, profit, advertising, market share, and so forth.

The definition of "quality" from a generic academic point of view may thus be looked at in view of philosophy, economics, marketing and likely with other secondary orientations. While *philosophers* may see quality in terms of universally recognizable innate excellence suggesting high standards and achievements, they normally consider the notion as undefinable in any precise terms and as something that can best be identified through experience. The issue is further complicated by associating quality with "beauty" which is inherently "logically primitive", which cannot be defined and which must be experienced in order to comprehend[5]. *Economists* have seen quality as something quite objective and measurable. A product's or service's quality is made up of the quality and quantity of its components, hence it can be compared and ranked. Quality is inherent, by way of the presence or absence of measurable product attributes within the product and not something attributed it. If the entire market, or a vast majority of it, considers the ranking acceptable, the quality definition then is decisive and unambiguous in contrast to situations where there are valid social or market-wide questions as to the acceptability of a product. Furthermore, much of the early research in economics associated quality with durability as it could in that fashion be easily incorporated into theoretical models. Higher quality was seen in terms of a longer stream of services emanating from the product hence easier measurability for model adaptation[6]. If a product is of higher quality, it contains more or better ingredients hence must command a correspondingly higher price. Indeed, quality differences may be reflected by way of, not necessarily proportional, shifts in the product's demand curve[7].

Finally, *marketing* people see quality as a form of perception in the eyes of the beholder. Thus, quality and quality ranking and relationships are perceived by the consumer. These rankings are achieved by the perceived presence of some combination of product attributes which provide the greatest level of consumer satisfaction[8]. On these premises, any product may look attractive and seem to be of higher quality. Appropriately intensive and persistent brainwashing and information manipulation can create a "high quality" product or even a high quality person. It may also be that if such perception creation campaigns are persistent enough, considerable difficulties may be encountered in trying to differentiate between the true quality of a product or service or simply the fact that consumers are accustomed to it, hence merely perceive it on that quality standard. This type of manipulative marketing is practiced in various sectors of the economy, and the professions including entertainment where intensively repeated customer exposure to certain "artists" through the media essentially brainwashes the consumer to think that they like the product instead of simply having become accustomed to it because of the product's contrived notoriety. In this fashion, the quality and marketability of the show, song, film, service, product or person becomes synonymous with the marketability of the entities involved. Once that is achieved, the entity becomes the marketable celebrity, and everything that happens to that "celebrity" including spontaneous or contrived trivial events of no social consequence even in his or her personal lives become a tool of merchandising. Thus, consumer perception is molded by the cooperation between various forms of media, marketing and agents. In this marketing jungle the true meaning, definition and measurability of quality become even more obscure, as it can simply be created or imagized by elaborate systems of public and private manipulation. These public relation gestures by way of selling and image-making efforts persist in many forms and in all types of markets, institutions, personal and organizational environments, indeed in all walks of life. It may be found in the hypothetical scenario of a Rambo-style administrator's relentless drive with huge opportunity costs to float a liberal arts-bred business program by way of the imagized credentials of some faculty, or that of a large industrial company's CEO aggressively imagizing his/her products in similarly competitive markets. They render the distinction between true quality and drummed-up myths and images rather obscure.

Under these circumstances it becomes all but impossible to aggregate varying individual preferences so as to create a meaningful market definition or measurement of product quality. The difficulty may at least nominally be overcome by appealing to population or market consensus as to certain product or service attributes, assuming that all individuals attach the same importance to those quality attributes in the first place, supported by unbiased statistical procedures aimed at aggregating preferences, disregarding differences in weights given by consumers to various quality attributes or to quality attributes all together. Thus, when economists depict quality changes simply by shifting the demand curve which incorporates a summation of individual preferences without explaining how that demand curve was derived in the first place, they simply disregard this aggregation problem[9].

In addition, even without the convoluted and contrived marketing environments discussed above, the distinction between the ingredients of true product quality and those factors which simply increase or even maximize consumer satisfaction all but disappears. Although the notions of product quality and consumer satisfaction may be related, they are not the same.

Some of the Basic Elements of Product Quality

Under the above described circumstances the task of delineating objective dimensions and elements of product quality becomes quite difficult, although not impossible. Some analysts have touched upon the subject in the past but most of the literature appears to have circumnavigated the subject[10]. Product or service *performance*, the primary operating attributes of the product or service, may be one such element of quality. However, while this attribute may be used for product or service ranking, it may be up to an individual consumer to associate product performance with quality itself, based upon the consumer's own expectations of specific performance dimensions. Diversity may dominate in perception of quality. Furthermore, performance may not be indicative of quality at all if it suggests a product category (e.g. a more powerful stereo amplifier putting out louder sounds does not necessarily suggest a quality superior to a less powerful one).

Product *attributes* may also be an element of quality, although less substantive than performance (e.g. leather instead of synthetic material seats in cars). Once again, consumer perception may or may not make this element decisive in terms of quality. In healthcare, a perennially smiling white-haired physician projecting a fatherly figure may have traditionally been associated by an unassuming patient with the provider of a better healthcare quality rather than with simply a form of product "packaging". On the other hand, in the medical sector, a physician with the same cozy personality and disposition may indeed in some respects be able to deliver a higher quality of healthcare, if his or her disposition is perceived by the patient as comforting and fulfills at least the psychological dimensions of patient-physician interaction. The overall quality of healthcare delivered by the physician would of course depend on the overall health status outcome of the patient after the treatment, and the latter is likely to depend not only on the physician's personality, perceived by the patient or otherwise, but also on his or her technical competence, experience, and propensity to keep up with the current research and literature relevant to the practice.

While it may be considered a part of performance, product *durability, reliability and serviceability* are also elements of quality but with an important time dimension such as the frequency of product failures and the need for servicing during a time period or in time intervals, and the length of time a product can remain in actual use (i.e. useful life). In medicine this is more likely to apply to therapeutic equipment such as tools of radiology (x-rays, ultrasound, cat scan, MRIs etc.). In some respects, durability correlates with serviceability as the latter will likely extend the former. The undertaking of service in order to extend the useful life of a product clearly depends on the cost of service in relation to the cost of replacement with a new product and the reliability and useful life extension that the service can expect to generate. The durability, serviceability and reliability of the product may all be determined in turn by utilization intensity and may very well vary inversely with the latter. Consequently, when we examine the causal relationships among the former three factors we normally assume that utilization intensity remains constant.

An interesting product/service quality element, also from a healthcare point of view, may be *conformance* to some set standards. In product manufacturing sectors, this element is simply the extent to which a product meets specific established standards from the beginning of its useful life, and in view of the frequency of needed repairs. Thus, conformance may be seen as a close cousin of reliability, although in some cases more extensive than reliability: failure in the latter will likely cause the product to cease effective functioning, while the former may be violated in minor manners which may cause interference with meeting set specific product standards but does not interfere with the effective utilization of the product, although it might alter related marketing practices (e.g. tires with and without blemishes).

In the medical service delivery sector conformance takes on added significance. Indeed, a major, often the most significant, yardstick for quality measurements or deviations from quality standards are conformance or lack thereof to community standards for practicing medicine. Much of a typical medical malpractice drama played out during pre-trial discovery and at trial centers on whether or not the provider(s) in delivering medical care conformed to established community standards for practice in the disputed care area. While the comparison with community standards of practice is a relatively objective process, the delineation and interpretation of the basis of the comparison, that is the community standard itself, may take on substantial subjective dilemmas.

We may look at one more element of quality, one that is quite subjective in nature, namely that of consumer *cognition*. These include the application of the consumer's personal judgment in terms of appearance, sound, and so forth, depending on the product. Our earlier discussion regarding the media's extensive manipulation of consumer tastes in order to "force" the acceptability of products, services, performers, certain performances, and even public figures by way of intensive advertising which are often tantamount to outright campaigning is clearly relevant here. So is our earlier reference in this chapter to the smiling white mustached and ever smiling fatherly physician who, while he may not be quite up to date with current research and the literature or even skill level applications, can certainly project a fine image of competence, generate psychological dependence and trust in the patient, and even benefit from a positive marketing fall-out by patient generated verbal advertising in friendship and family circles. However, we did indicate also that the psychological comfort induced by this type of provider in his or her patient may itself be beneficial, provided such comfort does not lull the patient into a "confidence trap" to the point where the patient should, but does not, seek alternative opinions or treatments.

Cognition may actually interfere with objective efforts to assess quality. Thus, objective efforts to rank academic departments within a discipline among universities based on articles published in leading journals by department faculty may have been tempered by subjective perceptions generated by the universities' historical reputation and prestige[11]. Similar subjective predicaments may be encountered when comparing private and institutional healthcare providers. A university with a better overall reputation than another is almost always assumed in the community to have a better medical school, clinics and treating physicians even if at times that may not be the case. In addition, the intensity of locally targeted advertising by hospitals, clinics and physician groups can further confuse patient perceptions of relative and absolute care quality levels.

The Industrial Economics of Quality

There are several major economic variables which are either determined by quality, or themselves determine quality, or both. That is, the relationship between quality and some other economic variables may under some circumstances be unilateral, and be under other circumstances bilateral. The most often considered economic variable in relation to quality is *price*. Given sufficient information at the disposal of consumers to assess the quality of a product or service, the usual postulate assumes a positive relationship between quality and price, where quality is thought to have come about at higher costs, and the latter in turn brings about the higher price. Lacking adequate information to assess quality, consumers may attempt to make informed judgment regarding at least relative quality by comparing prices, with the presumption that the higher the price of a comparable product the higher must its quality be. The price-quality relationship is seen as positive with the causation running from price to quality, instead of the normal fundamental notion of quality, through costs, determine price. Thus, this reversal of the perceived relationship direction between quality and price can prompt producers to increase profits by simply increasing price (with or without prompting a reduction in costs to further increase profits) and enhancing the quality image of the product without actually increasing or even possibly maintaining quality. The price quality relationship gets distorted and becomes even negative[12].

Some empirical studies in this area appear to find a similar lack of consistency. A number of studies found the traditional and consistent positive correlation between price and quality[13], while some others found inconsistent results, depending on whether the product was durable or nondurable, with the former demonstrating positive relationships between price and quality and the latter negative[14]. In fact, where other market elements such as brand name, image, or even country of origin, are introduced the bilateral relationship, negative or positive and in either direction, between price and quality becomes obscured and may even virtually disappear.

Another economic variable often examined in relation to quality is direct *production cost*. The relationship is quite complex and the literature is by no means consistent in its nature. One obvious thought would have the two variables as positively related based on the assumption that quality depends on its various elements, discussed earlier, and the utilization of elements in a manner that will generate improved quality requires more or more expensive materials and additional labor hours in the production process yielding higher costs. Data surveys on the other hand presented a confusing picture. Thus, a survey in 1977 found that costs directly attributed to quality averaged around only 5-8% of sales depending largely on the quality control systems implemented[15].

Variations in cost-quality relationships by industry, reflecting in part on varied product quality definitions, have also been shown by studies based on the PIMS [Profit Impact of Marketing Strategies] database. Thus, a positive relationship was found in industries producing differentiated products and a negative one for those producing homogeneous goods. Positive relationship was demonstrated in capital goods producing industries but a negative one for those producing the components of capital goods[16].

Another interesting and less confusing quality-based relationship is that with *profitability*. Studies in general seem to point to a positive relationship between quality and profitability. One explanation rests with the decreased elasticity of demand for a product of higher quality, thus affording it an opportunity for selling at a higher price without much decrease in quantity demanded. The cost of attaining higher quality is more than offset by increased revenues. In addition, as quality increases by way of increasing the weight of quality elements discussed earlier, so does the cost of doing so but once again accompanied by a greater increase in revenue hence profitability[17]. Empirical studies utilizing the PIMS data also indicate that at same or similar levels of markets share there is a positive relationship between quality and profitability, the latter measured as return on investment[18].

The relationship between *advertising* and quality was found to be positive by some studies. The quality elements were embodied in two different categories of goods. The so called "search" product quality elements can be ascertained prior to purchase and use, while those of "experience" goods can be determined only after acquisition and use. It was in fact argued that for experienced goods persistent advertising does generate higher product quality perceptions particularly when such advertising belabors quality issues[19].

Other studies have disputed this positive relationship. A relatively recent consumer survey as well as some other studies yielded no particular relationship between quality by way of perceived dependability and advertising[20].

The relationship between quality and product *market-share* is tempered by the price of the product itself. During any specific time period, holding other contributory factors constant, the volume of sales is a function of price. The relative and absolute volume of sales in turn is a major determinant of market share. To enhance quality, more of its elements need to be embodied in the product, generating higher costs, hence higher price. Thus, if quality is defined in terms of the number of its elements present, the relationship between quality and market share is likely to be negative. If, on the other hand, quality is seen merely in terms of one element such as suitability, or conformance to some standard, or aesthetics, then the cost of attaining any one of these elements need not be high, hence nor do prices. In that even, quality (as a selling incentive) and market-share may show a positive relationship. Empirical studies in general appear to have pointed to a similar positive relationship between quality and market share[21].

Quality clearly has different interpretations in different economic sectors and industries. The quality of a pair of shoes needs to be examined in terms of different dimensions than that of a car, or that of a healthcare service. We already noted that quality is a multi-dimensional concept where the number of dimensions, the composition of the dimensions, and the relevant time dimensions differ by the type of product or service under consideration. Furthermore, in addition to the number, composition and timing of the dimensions, various intra-quality-dimensional relationships (IQDRs) among the various quality dimensions for any product or service need also be examined, a task which may empirically be quite difficult. Thus, from examining the notion of quality even in a generic context, it continues to appear to be an elusively difficult concept to deal with, to define and to measure. The flow of literature as well as ideas is likely to continue for the time being, particularly in the healthcare sector where the complexities are compounded by the complex nature of the product and service themselves, of the production, distribution, consumption process, and related payment or regulatory systems.

Another Look at Quality in an Industrial Setting - Deming in a Nutshell

W. Edward Deming's name has often been associated with the successful development of the post-war Japanese economy, and while historically revered in that country, he was largely disregarded in post-war United States, particularly during the first decades of the post-war period when the US economy seemed invincible both domestically and on the international scene. The US having the only undamaged manufacturing structure in the world could do nothing wrong economically at that time. Deming theories were not needed here, but were welcomed by the Japanese in their efforts to reconstruct their country and economy. Quality was not an important US manufacturing consideration. The main preoccupation at that time was with meeting domestic and world-wide demand. The issue of quality, and Deming's criteria for manufacturing success, fell through the cracks of production quotas and almost automatic and self-generating prosperity.

Not having met much recognition by top management in the US during early 1905, Deming accepted an invitation by the Japanese industry leaders. The latter were concerned with Japan's image - at that time - as a manufacturer of inferior products. Deming's seminar series and involvement in quality related decisions and processes at the top management level was apparently the catalyst in Japan's turn-around into a manufacturer of high quality product and the corresponding change in its image.

A Ph.D. in physics, Deming's theories are presented in terms of fourteen broad criteria which may be applicable not only in manufacturing but also in the service industries, including healthcare. The general theme centers on Total Quality Management (TQM) which is a collective name for quality enhancement through statistical methods. These fourteen criteria may be used as a checklist for organizations wishing to improve the quality of their product or service, and may very briefly be summed up as follows: (a) the purpose of product or service quality improvement is consistent and constant; (b) a philosophy of learning from past mistakes is adopted; (c) instead of relying on mass inspection procedures, the production process itself needs to be improved, and to verify that a 100% inspection may need to be implemented; (d) purchasing decisions rely mainly on quality and not price, or if price then are subject to quality constraints, with provisions for readily accommodated product adjustment; (e) quality improvement is viewed as a dynamic and perennial process concentrating on quality at the production level instead of follow-up scrutiny; (f) the system should provide for adequate training of product/service producers, training which should be viewed as an extension of product/service quality; (g) management should be familiar with employee job circumstances, and can be without necessarily having the skills of the employees involved; (h) the workplace should be free of fear and feelings of insecurity, particularly those often related to possible suggestions and other contributions that employees may make; (i) cross-sectional team-work by way of multi-managerial level committees prevent breakdown of communications, misunderstandings, and hostilities; (j) avoid unrealistic targets, such as zero error requirements and demands for perfection; (k) quantity quotas are counter-productive, intimidating, and ultimately may also be constraining; (l) promptly meet employees' need for approval wherever warranted, and minimize status barriers to effective communications; (m) secure favorable conditions for perpetual retraining and education; and finally, (n) impose and impress quality related doctrines and convictions on top management first, and then on middle and lower management[22].

Structure, Process and Outcome Revisited

We have already noted that healthcare quality is a function of a large number of independent and interdependent variables. Nonetheless, three major dimensions of quality have now been consistently accepted as base criteria for defining and assessing healthcare quality: structure, process and outcome[23]. Scholars have included a variety of quality criteria under *structural* considerations. In general, these comprise the settings and conditions under which healthcare is delivered. More specifically, quality criteria such as adequate (in terms of quality and quantity) staffing, staff attitudes and training levels, patient environment (patient room conditions), effectiveness, efficiency, social acceptability, relevance to need, credibility, and competitiveness are among the major items included in this category[24].

Earlier efforts to view *process* related quality criteria centered on personal psychological care, group comfort situations, physical care, communication, professional responsibility allocation and adherence, and competence[25]. Subsequent studies in this regard concentrated first on the quality of care service recordings, based on the assumption that the quality of recording correlated with, and was an indicator of, the quality of the care given. The rationale was that care recording constituted the basis for further care evaluation and hence was the mirror of the care given[26]. Other works viewed quality in terms of the person providing the care rather than the care itself, placing the emphases on the interpersonal skill of the provider instead of just on performing care tasks. Thus, individualizing care becomes an important process element implemented by efforts such as extended listening to patients, providing emotional support and comfort, as well as consulting with family members[27].

Finally, care *outcome* related criteria refer to the health status of the patient after the process or a phase of it is complete. Indicators such as wellness, mortality, disease, disability, discomfort, dissatisfaction, etc. can all be used (as we will particularly note in the next two chapters) to assess care outcome. In general, outcome may be viewed as an alteration in the health status of the patient, and when seen in terms of some desired quality that alteration is presumed to some degree to be positive. Thus, outcome is seen as a contributing component of quality, and may be viewed or assessed in a number of terms such as physiology, psychology, service frequency, need(s) to rehospitalize or reinstitutionalize, costs, symptom control, diagnostic effectiveness and so forth[28]. These issues will be taken up in detail in the following two chapters

General Healthcare Quality Symptoms

Before embarking on a detailed examination of specific healthcare quality related issues, in particular definitions, measurements and assessments, I review here some of the general criteria which have often been used to assess healthcare quality both in institutional and private provider settings. Much of these criteria are predicated upon fear and control generated by third-party payment policies, cost consciousness, and constrained financial incentives for individual and institutional providers, to minimize costs, maximize profits, and at the expense of quality. The US Government (HCFA) has attempted to disseminate some information regarding care quality by way of hospital specific mortality rates experienced by Medicare beneficiaries since 1986. We will look at this type of data later. Suffice it to say here that the effort received much criticism due to alleged data gathering and interpretation problems and the consequent dissemination of apparently misleading information. Since mid-1988, the Office of Technology Assessment (OTA) began looking at some medical care quality indicators that could be useful for enhancing informed consumer choice[29].

The various quality criteria developed by the OTA must be seen in terms of some inherent and by no means about to be solved problems, related mostly to inherent complexities of the care process, the difficulty in measuring psychological elements, interpersonal relationships, and the varied dimensions of the application of the technical aspects of medical science and technology, not mentioning legitimate variations in practice styles, and the varied interpretation of already published care related studies that remain controversial with a significant proportion of practitioners, such as the relationship between cholesterol and heart disease, cholesterol and diet in contrast to genetic dispositions, the relationship between fat and various diseases such as colo-rectal and breast cancer, just to mention a few[30]. The various interpretations of and attitudes to published studies, and the perceived biases instilled by the financial sponsors of the studies (legend has it that the studies which showed correlation between eggs and high blood cholesterol, thus the implications of otherwise highly nutritious eggs in connection to heart disease, was financed by the cereal industry) often necessitate indispensable reliance on so called standards, generated by medical consensus.

Universally accepted standards for medical practice have been hard to come by. These standards are sought after as yardsticks for various performance indicators. If the standards are not there, then the association among the various quality indicators may need to be relied upon. Yet, quality indicators themselves may be drastically different and the reasoning somewhat circuitous. Thus, for instance, the presence of the already discussed quality indicators in the *structural* category (such as organizational arrangements and available resources for care delivery) may be viewed as permitting better performance, while their absence might be a source for concern, might also allow an analyst to consider the extent to which these structural factors by themselves contribute to quality as distinct from the provider's contribution. In other words could the same provider perform just as well under less favourable structural environments, or could a less competent provider perform better under a better structural environment than a poorer one. What proportion of the performance improvement may be attributed to the environment and what proportion to the provider? A correct answer to these questions would go a long way toward more efficient resource allocation. In addition, the dilemma leads us right into considering the other care category, namely the *process* of care (the activities of providers providing care), which, as we saw above, may not be readily separated from structure in the first place. Yet, even with process related considerations one might argue that efficient resource allocation might dictate a selective scrutiny of performance episodes focusing only on those which have been shown to substantially improve or notably harm patients. If so, then we find ourselves right in the area of the third general set of performance criteria, also discussed before, namely care *outcome* that entails quality measurements in terms of provider yielded health status. As we noted earlier, however, this is also muddy territory, for emerging health status and satisfaction of a patient may be influenced, indeed determined, to various extents by several factors other than, or in addition to, the services directly generated by the provider. The upshot of this analytical labyrinth may be that these three overlapping sets of quality measurement criteria should be viewed not as alternative measurements but rather closely related complements for, or supplements to, each other. Process as a measure of quality must be associated with patient outcome, and patient outcome in turn must be related to a significant extent to some previously performed process, while both of these need to be specifically related to some specific elements of the structural environment[31]. Notwithstanding these issues, let us take a quick look at some possible quality indicators in institutional, private provider, and payment system settings.

HCFA has been routinely publishing *hospital mortality* data, although there does not appear to have been any serious efforts made to scrutinize these mortality analyses[32]. VA hospitals run by the Veterans Administration have also been evaluated in terms of their mortality rates, but apparently with more scrutiny as the VA has examined the records of low and high mortality rate hospitals with a view to validation proceedings[33]. In general, some questions were raised about the reliability of the data used in mortality studies, and problems in discharge data as well as in uniform data coding and collections were identified[34].

In addition, other studies cautioned of the possible flaws with mortality data as a yardstick of healthcare quality. One study of above average mortality hospitals in New York State found serious quality problems in no more than 3% of those hospitals. Another study has found fewer quality problems in high mortality hospitals than in other ones[35]. PROs conducted a review of hospitals with various mortality rates and found no significant care difference among 56% of these institutions, and not enough information with much of the rest of them[36]. Yet, when adjusting hospital mortality rates for patient risk of dying and pre-existing conditions, another study found that preventable mortality occurred with a higher frequency in high-mortality institutions than in low ones[37].

A care quality symptom somewhat akin to mortality although clearly not as severe is the frequency of various negative events, such as nosocomial infections, that may occur in an institution per some time period, say a year. In order for these events to be considered quality indicators, they clearly need to be separated from other patient characteristics and risk factors. Furthermore, since reporting practices and systems vary, a high frequency of reported negative events in a hospital may in fact be an indicator of *better* rather than poorer quality of care due to a possibly better system of scrutiny and reporting in place in the higher reporting institution than in the one reporting a lower incidence, as the actual but unreported frequency of these events in the latter may in fact be higher.

Disciplinary actions and sanctions implemented or recommended by PROs, the Department of Health and Human Services and state medical boards may be seen as a category of quality indicators. At an assumed level of rigor, these may be suggestive of the quality of the providers involved. Yet, their utility may be quite limited. For instance, some half of the disciplinary actions taken against physicians were related to writing prescriptions[38], while essential to good care, clearly not a pivotal point for its assessment. Most of the other actions against physicians were alcohol or other drug abuse related. In addition, while state sanctioned providers are clearly identified (although the information is not always readily communicated or even available to consumers), not all physicians with quality problems, but unsanctioned, are likely to be identified[39]. On the other hand, HCFA has leverage over care quality provided to Medicare patients through PROs. These reviews do cover incompetent or inappropriate care, and problems with documentation; the latter may not be indicative of poor care, but nor is it conducive for ascertaining quality care.

Another possible area of quality scrutinization may under some circumstances be within the realm of *medical malpractice litigation*, verdicts, judgments and awards, although questionably settlements. An immediate problem with using this category is its extremely limited scope within the patient population since no more than about 1% of those who may have been harmed actually file a medical malpractice claim, and even among those that have been litigated there may be a substantial proportion which did not actually involve any significant malfeasance by the provider[40]. In addition, a single incident of malpractice may or may not reflect on the provider's competence, although repeated claims against an individual may be an indication of a problem.

The amount of the jury award itself is probably irrelevant to quality assessment, since those awards include a variety compensation elements related mostly to the nature of the injury and compensable losses sustained by the claimant, such as pain and suffering, future medical expenses, loss of earning capacity, and the like the compensation for which is far removed from the nature of the original malfeasance by the provider; unless, claims for punitive damages are sustained by a jury based on by its having been persuaded by plaintiff's counsel that the provider was grossly negligent. However, even punitive damages may be viewed with skepticism as a yardstick of the malfeasance and negative quality, since the amount of the punitive damage award is largely dependent on the relative skill of the attorneys involved as well as on the subjective assessment and perceptions by the jurors and their sympathies for the claimant, hardly a scientifically supportable or particularly measurable notion.

Another problem with using medical malpractice litigation as a quality indicator is that many, if not most, cases actually settle, prior to the verdict stage of the trial, or even before the commencement of the trial. The settlement amount is, once again, dependent on the actors involved. The legal profession is colorful and highly heterogeneous. Some plaintiff attorneys with limited or undistinguished trial experience or competence in the field, while motivated financially to take on a medical malpractice case, do so with a predisposition to settlement rather than trying it in order to obtain possibly the maximum compensation for their client. The rationale normally expressed is in terms of the "risks" and "uncertainties" involved in a trial and the unpredictability of a jury. These elements, to be sure, are indeed present in all jury trials, however, their potential negative impact on the outcome of the case from the victim's point of view varies inversely with the quality, experience, diligence and conscientiousness of plaintiff's counsel. For some plaintiff's attorneys, the perceived marginal cost (in preparation, extra work and possibly training and a variety of other terms) of developing and preparing a case for trial is far greater than the marginal revenue (in view of some mathematical expectation) by way of the additional fees that a verdict larger than the settlement might generate. Thus, once again, the amount of the settlement may be more indicative of the relative competence, work propensities and proclivities of the lawyers, and to some extent the personality of their client, than the nature and extent of the medical malfeasance involved. In addition, medical malpractice suits have also been shown to reflect the patient's dissatisfaction only in terms of the care's interpersonal aspects rather than its technical quality[41].

Even successful malpractice claims need to be viewed in terms of the specialities, patient risks and likely potential outcomes for the patients involved, before physician profiles regarding care quality can be conclusively drawn. Other factors, such as physician case-loads and patient-mix also need to be looked at prior to assessing care quality based on medical malpractice litigation. Finally, looking at physician malpractice profiles over long-enough time periods to permit some reliability in care quality conclusions would also be advisable. An isolated claim against a physician, even if successful, may not conclusively indicate technical care deficiency. Once again, factors such as relative legal skills and artificial jury perceptions could play an important role. However, a number of successful or even settled claims against the same provider should be a cause for serious further inquiries.

External standards and evaluations have long been a part of the quality assessment scene. While not considered as the ultimate assurance of optimum quality, compliance with external standards does appear to suggest the availability and utilization of adequate quantity and quality of resources by a hospital to perform its scope of functions. Such frequently applied external accreditation is one by the Joint Commission on the Accreditation of Healthcare Organizations (JCAHO). The JCAHO in its accreditation procedures evaluates virtually all aspects of a hospital's operations, and since it does accredit a vast majority of the hospitals it looks at, those few that do fail its tests might provide valid grounds for professional care quality scrutiny.

Perhaps the most important automatic indicator of quality, by itself and even better used along with other indicators such as mortality rates, is the *volume of services performed*, particularly for hospitals. The performance experience factor (PEF). Studies have found a positive relationship between low PEFs in *hospital* acute care environments, such as cardiac surgery, and a higher incidence of mortality or negative patient outcomes. However, PEF was found to be a less convincing quality indicator for private practitioners[42]. Once again, the relationship between volume and outcome, even in a hospital environment, needs to be assessed in the light of patient-mix and other risk factors, and be examined over several years, instead of just one year.

PEF for physicians may closely be linked to fields of practice endeavors. Physicians practice in a certain field either because they were originally trained in that field or because they have, by virtue of meeting other performance criteria, received speciality board certification in that field. Studies suggest that training is a stronger indicator of physician potential performance quality than speciality board certification, although the impact of patient-physician interpersonal relationships was not considered[43]. The impact of that relationship need not distort patient perceptions (positive or negative) of care quality even regarding the technical aspects of care in ambulatory care situations, although those perceptions do not seem as reliable in more involved technical, particularly inpatient, care processes[44]. Clearly, patient perceptions may very well be distorted by various subjective relational factors which may or may not have anything to do with the technical aspects of the care.

Furthermore, the development of standardized data (beyond rudimentary opinion surveys) may be a difficult task to adequately accomplish. The Agency for Health Policy and Research, created recently by the Omnibus Budget Reconciliation Act of 1989[45], could have been the way to solve the standardized and appropriate data generation problem. Much of the published data, for instance, address the patient's condition at discharge. However, discharge data does not indicate the condition of the patient at the time of admission, or the structure and process of care that was applied to that condition, so that quality can be assessed not only in the light of outcome but also in terms of the various care elements that led to that outcome. Once again, the significance of the multilateral relationships among the previously discussed three stages of care assessment (structure-process-outcome) become relevant. Discharge data addresses patient status only after the administration of care, and cannot address the need for and propriety of that care in view of the patient's condition at the time of admittance and during inpatient status. In ambulatory settings (physicians' offices), even discharge data is often difficult to obtain, and the researcher may need to resort to claims submitted to third-party payers to generate some type of relevant data, even if they may not contain the clinical details necessary to assess the quality of care delivered. Clearly, an area that requires much more work.

Finally, even if proper data are generated, such data have functions beyond that which enable researchers to properly assess healthcare quality, namely, to inform and educate consumers. Hence, effective dissemination of proper data to the public is important. Efforts in that regard also appear to be in a relatively infantile stage, and vary state-by-state. Thus, since the mid-1980s New York State has required hospitals to report negative occurrences to the state Department of Health, which are subsequently used to generate periodic reports, although without naming the hospitals involved. Similar efforts have been implemented in Massachusetts where HMOs, clinics and hospitals are required to submit information regarding certain negative occurrences to the Office of Consumer Affairs. Specific physicians are involved in some states' reporting system. Pennsylvania publicly disseminates physician-specific information regarding quality, and Arizona releases physician-specific patient discharge data. Most of the other states which also collect similar data, do not release physician-specific information[46]. This is likely to change in future years as cost and quality consciousness increasingly pervades the healthcare consuming population.

Notes

1. Leathard, A., "Crisis in the NHS: Lessons from Home and Abroad" in *Health Care Provision: Past, Present and Future*, Chapman and Hall, London, 1990.
2. Fetter, R.B., Freeman, J.L., "Diagnosis Related Group: A Product Oriented Approach to Hospital Management" in Fetter, R.B., Thompson, J.D., Kimberly, J.R., *Cases in Health Policy Management*, Richard D. Irwin, Homewood IL, 1985, pp. 229-51.
3. Donabedian, A., "The Quality of Care: How Can it be Assessed?" in Grahan, N.O., *Quality Assurance in Hospitals.*, Hospital Administration Press, 1990, pp. 14-28.
4. Freeman, J.L., Duncan, C.C., Fetter, R.B., *Beyond DRGs: Patient Classification for Episodes of Care*, Proceedings of the 7th International PCS/E Working Conference, 1991; II: 22-27.
5. Pirsig, R.M., *Zen and the Art of Motorcycle Maintenance*, Bantam Books, New York, 1974. See also Tuchman, B.W., "The Decline of Quality", *The New York Times Magazine*, November 2, 1980. Buchanen, S. (ed), *The Portable Plato*, Viking Press, New York, 1948. Dickie, G., *Aesthetics: An Introduction*, The Bobbs-Merril Co. Inc., New York, 1971.
6. Abbott, L., *Quality and Competition*, Columbia University Press, New York, 1955. Lancaster, K., *Consumer Demand: A new Approach*, Columbia University Press, New York, 1971. See also Lancaster, L., *Variety, Equity and Efficiency*, Columbia University Press, New York, 1979. Leffer, K.B., "Ambiguous Changes in Product Quality", *American Economic Review*, December 1982. Griliches, Z. (ed), *Price Indexes and Quality Change*, Harvard University Press, Cambridge MA, 1971. Lehvari, D., and Srinivasan, T.N., "Durability of Consumption Goods: Competition v. Monopoly", *American Economic Review*, March 1969. Saving, T.R., "Market Organization and Product Quality", *Southern Economic Journal*, April 1982. Swan, P.L., "Durability of Consumer Goods", *American Economic Review*, December 1970. Schmalensee, R.L., "Regulation and the Durability of Goods", *Bell Journal of Economics and Management Science*, Spring 1970.
7. Chamberlin, E.H., "The Product as an Economic Variable", *Quarterly Journal of Economics*, February 1953. See also Dorfman, R., Steiner, P.O., "Optimal Advertising and Optimal Quality", *American Economic Review*, December 1954; and White, L.J., "Quality Variations When Prices are Regulated", *Bell Journal of Economics and Management Science*, Fall 1972.
8. Kuehn, A.A. and Day, R.L., "Strategy of Product Quality", *Harvard Business Review*, November 12, 1962
9. Edwards, C., "The Meaning of Quality", *Quality Progress* , October 1968. Theil, H., *Principles of Econometrics*, John Wiley & Sons Inc, New York, 1971, pp. 556-73; and Sheshinski, E., "Price, Quality and Quantity Regulation in a Monopoly Situation", *Economica*, May 1976.
10. Juran, J.M. (ed), *Quality Control Handbook*, 3rd Ed., McGraw-Hill, New York, 1974. Also see Maynes, E.S., "The Concept and Management of Product Quality" in Terleckyj, N.E. (ed), *Household Production and Consumption*, National Bureau of Economic Research, New York, 1976, pp. 529-60.
11. Hagstrom, W.O., "Inputs, Outputs and the Prestige of American University Science Departments", *Sociology of Education*, Fall 1971. Knudsen, D.D., Vaughan, T.R., "Quality in Graduate Education: A Re-Evaluation of Rankings of Sociology Departments in the Carter Report", *American Sociologist*, February 1969.

12. Lambert, D.R., "Price as a Quality Signal: The Tip of the Iceberg", *Economic Inquiry*, 1980. See also Riesz, P.C., "The Price Quality Relations for Packaged Foods Products", *Journal of Consumer Affairs*, Winter 1979.

13. McConnell, J.D., "An Experimental Examination of Price-Quality Relationships", *Journal of Business*, October 1968. See also Gabor, A., Granger, C.W.J., "Price as an Indicator of Quality: Report on an Enquiry", *Economica*, February 1966.

14. Riesz, P.C. 1979; and Westbrook, R.A., Newman, J.W., Taylor, J.R., "Satisfaction/Dissatisfaction in the Purchase Decision Process", *Journal of Marketing*, October 1978.

15. "Quality Cost Survey", *Quality*, June 1977. See also Crosby, P.B., *Quality is Free*, New York, 1979, and by the same author "Product Performance Cost", *Quality Progress*, June 1974 and Gilmore, H.L., "Consumer Product Quality Control Costs Revisited", *Quality Progress*, April 1983.

16. Gale, B.T. and Branch, B.S., "Concentration v Market Share: Which Determines Performance and Why Does it Matter", *The Antitrust Bulletin*, Spring 1982, pp. 82-105; see also Phillips, L.W., Chang, D., Buzzell, R.D., "Product Quality, Cost Position and Business Performance: A Test of Some Key Hypotheses", *Journal of Marketing*, Spring 1983, pp. 26043.

17. Chamberlin, E.H., "The Product as Economic Variable", *Quarterly Journal of Economics*, February 1953, pp. 1-23. See also Dorfman, R., Steiner, P.O., "Optimal Advertising and Optimal Quality", *American Economic Review*, December 1954.

18. Craig, C.S. and Douglas, S.P. "Strategic Factors Associated with Market and Financial Performance", *Quarterly Review of Economics and Business*, Summer 1982. Also Phillip, Chang and Buzzell (1983), and Schoeffler, S., Buzzell, R.D. and Henry, D.F., "Impact of Strategic Planning on Profit Performance", *Harvard Business Review*, March-April 1974.

19. Nelson, P., "Information and Consumer Behavior", *Journal of Political Economy*, March 1970, and Scmalensee, R.L., "A Model of Advertising and Product Quality", *Journal of Political Economy*, June 1978.

20. Barksdale, H.C., Perreault, W.D., et al., "A Cross National Survey of Consumer Attitudes Towards Marketing Practices, Consumerism and Government Regulations", *Columbia Journal of World Business*, Summer 1982. See also Rotfeld, H.J. and Rozol, K.B., "Advertising and Product Quality: Are Heavily Advertised Products Better?", *Journal of Consumer Affairs*, September 1976; Gilligan, C.T. and Holmes, D.E.A., "Advertising Expenditure and Product Quality", *Management Decision*, Vol. 17, No. 5, pp. 393-403.

21. Buzzell, R.D. and Wiersema, F.D., "Successful Share Building Strategies", *Harvard Business Review*, January-February 1981. Buzzell, R.D. and Wiersema, F.D., "Modelling Changes in Market Share: A Cross Sectional Analysis", *Strategic Management Journal*, 1981. Gale, B.T. and Branch, B.S., "Concentration vs Market Share: Which Determines Performance and Why Does it Matter?", *The Antitrust Bulletin*, Spring 1982.

22. Deming, E.W., *Out of the Crisis*, MIT Center for Advanced Engineering Studies, Cambridge MA, 1986.

23. Donabedian, A., "Some Issues in Evaluating the Quality of Nursing Care", *American Journal of Public Health*, Vol. 59, 1966.

24. Bennett, A., "Quality of Care: Bridging the Gap Between Promise and Performance", *Trustee*, Vol. 37, No. 10, 1984. See also Maxwell, J.R., "Quality Assessment in Health", *British Medical Journal*, Vol. 288, 1984; Kitson, A., "Indicators of Quality in Nursing Care - An Alternative Approach", *Journal of Advance Nursing*,

Vol. 11, 1986; Jackson-Frankl, M.A., "The Language and Meaning of Quality", *Nursing Administration Quarterly,* Vol. 14, No. 3, 1990.

25.   Wandelt, M. and Stewart, D.S., *The Slater Nursing Competencies Rating Scale.* Appleton-Century-Crofts, New York, 1975; Felton, G., Frevert, E., Galligan, K., et al, "Implementation of Quality Assurance Program", *Journal of Nursing Administration,* Vol. 6, No. 1, 1976; Hagen, E., "Appraising the Quality of Nursing Care", *Nursing Research Conference,* Vol. 8, 1976. See also note 26.

26.   Wandelt, M. and Ager, J., *Quality Patient Care,* Appleton-Century-Crofts, New York, 1974; Jelink, R., Haussmann, R., Hegyvary, S., Newman, J., *Methodology for Monitoring the Quality of Care,* US Dept Health Education and Welfare, Bethesda MD, 1974.

27.   Donabedian, A., "Criteria, Norms and Standards of Quality - What Do They Mean", *American Journal of Public Health,* Vol. 71, No. 4, 1980. See also Parish, S., "Quality v Quantity: Which Type of Nursing Do You Practice?", *Journal of Practical Nursing,* Vol. 36, No. 2 1986, Valentine, K., "Caring in More than Kindness: Modeling Its Complexities", *Journal of Nursing Administration,* Vol. 11, No. 11, 1989, and Taylor, A., Hudson, K., Keeling, A., "Quality Nursing Care: The Consumers Perspective Revisited", *Journal of Nursing Quality Assurance,* Vol. 5, No. 2, 1991.

28.   Lohr, K., "Outcome Measurements: Concepts and Questions", *Inquiry,* Vol. 25, 1988. See also Zimmer, M., "Symposium on Quality Assurance", *Nursing Clinics of North America,* Vol. 9, No. 2, 1974; Rutstein et al, "Measuring the Quality of Medical Care", *New England Journal of Medicine,* Vol. 294, No. 11, 1976; Marek, K., "The Measurement of Patient Outcomes", *Journal of Nursing Quality Assurance,* Vol. 4, No. 3, 1989.

29.   US Department of Health and Human Services, Office of the Inspector General, Office of Analysis and Inspections, *Medical Licensure and Discipline: An Overview,* Washington, DC, 1986. US Congress, Office of Technology Assessment, *The Quality of Medical Care: Information for Consumers,* USGPO, Washington, DC, 1988.

30.   Atkins, R.C., *Dr. Atkins' New Diet Revolutions,* Evans & Co., New York, 1993. See also by the same author *Dr. Atkis' Health Revolution: How Complementary Medicine Can Extend Your Life,* Bantam Books, New York, 1988.

31.   These issues are examined further in Donabedian, A., "Evaluating the Quality of Medical Care", *Milbank Quartely,* Vol. 44, 1966, No. 3 part 2; the same author "Explorations in Quality Assessment and Monitoring" in *The Definition of Quality and Approaches to Its Assessment,* Vol. I, Health Administration Press, Ann Arbor MI, 1980. McAuliffe, W., "Studies of Process-Outcome Correlation in Medical Care Evaluations", *Medical Care,* Vol. 16, No. 11, 1978. Also see Brook, R.H., and Lohr, K.N., "Efficacy, Effectiveness, Variations and Quality", *Medical Care ,* Vol. 23, No. 51985.

32.   US Congress, General Accounting Office, *Medicare: An Assessment of HCFA's 1988 Hospital Mortality Analyses,* Washington, DC, US Govt Printing Office, 1988.

33.   US Congress, Office of Technology Assessment, *Assessment of Veterans Administration's Method of Analyzing its Hospital Mortality Rates,* Washington, DC, 1989.

34.   Demlo, L.K., Campbell, P.M. and Brown, S.S., "Reliability of Information Abstracted From Patient Medical Records", *Medical Care,* Vol. 16, 1978. Hsia, D.C., Krushat, W.M., Fagat, A.B., "Accuracy of Diagnostic Coding for Medicare Patients Under the Prospective Payment System", *New England Journal of Medicine,* Vol. 318, No. 6, 1988.

35.   New York State Department of Health, Office of Health Systems Management,

Bureau of Healthcare Research, *Investigation of Quality of Care in Hospitals*, Albany, 1987, and Hannan, E.L., Yazici, A.A., *Critique of the 1987 HCFA Mortality Study Based on New York Data*, Office of Health Systems Management, Albany, 1988.

36. US Congress, General Accounting Office, *Medicare: Improved Patient Outcome Analyses Could Enhance Quality Assessment*, GPO, Washington, DC, 1988.

37. DuBois, R.W, Rodgers, W.H., Moxley, J.H., "Hospital Inpatient Mortality: Is it a Predictor of Quality?", *New England Journal of Medicine*, Vol. 317, No. 26, 1987.

38. US Department of Health and Human Services, Office of the Inspector General, Office of Analysis and Inspections, *Medical Licensure and Discipline: An Overview*, Washington, DC, 1986

39. A privately published source (from Ralph Nader's group) for problem physician identification has become popular, since it lists physicians by name, address, various other biographical and personal data, the disciplinary action taken, the reason for the action, and other information: Public Citizens Health Research Group Report, *10289 Questionable Doctors*, Washington, DC, 1993.

40. Harvard Medical Practice Study, *Patients, Doctors, and Lawyers: Medical Injury, Malpractice Litigation, and Patient Compensation in New York*, Report to the State of New York, Boston MA, 1990.

41. American Board of Medical Specialities, *Medical Speciality Certification and Related Matters*, Evanston IL, 1987.

42. Hannan, E.L., O'Donnel, J.F. et al., "Investigation of the Relationship Between Volume and Mortality for Surgical Procedures Performed in New York State Hospitals", *JAMA*, Vol. 262, 1989. See also Luft, H.S., Garnick, D.W., Mark, D., *Evaluating Research on the Use of Volume of Services Performed in Hospitals as an Indicator of Quality*, Contractor Document. Office of Technology Assessment US Congress, Washington, DC, 1987.

43. Palmer, R.H., Reilly, M.C., "Individual and Institutional Variables Which Serve as Indicators of Quality of Medical Care", *Medical Care*, Vol. 17, No. 7, 1979.

44. Ware, J.E., Davies, A.R., Rubin, H.R., *The Suitability of Consumer Assessments of Physician and Hospital Performance as Indicators of the Quality of Care*, Contractor Document. Office of Technology Assessment, US Congress, Washington, DC, 1987.

45. Incorporated the former National Center for Health Services Research and Health Care Technology Assessment.

46. New York State Department of Health, *Incident Reporting for Hospitals*. Health Facilities Series H-61, Albany, Sept 30, 1985. US Congress, Office of Technology Assessment, *Quality of Medical Care: Information for Consumers*, US Government Printing Office, Washington, DC, 1988. Larks, M., *Access to Health Data by State Health Data Organizations and Quality Assessors*, Contractor Document. US Congress Office of Technology Assessment, Washington, DC, 1987.

3 Definitions and Delineations of Healthcare Quality

For over a century, in fact, perhaps since the beginning of medical practice in its modern form in the US the setting and policing of medical care quality standards by already licensed practitioners have been vested within the circles of the providers themselves. This was consistent with the inherent definition of a "profession", any profession, itself which centers on the establishment and enforcement of its own standards. In contrast to other professions, however, medical standards have always been seen by the layman in scientifically elusive terms probably supported by competently procured and tested empirical data. Conventional medicine, in contrast to other health practitioners (such as chiropractors, osteopath, homeopaths, etc.) was thus promoted or presented as science-based areas of endeavor thereby differentiating itself from all other similar disciplines. The presented scientific orientation of the discipline also generated an impression within and outside the medical profession to the effect that standards and quality can be defined and measured with greater rigor than in other fields of endeavor. This enhanced scientific rigor of care quality definition and measurement was accepted by society. In fact it had to be accepted by society, in the same time as medicine as a whole and its individual members succeeded at maintaining an unusually high level of professional autonomy, set their own working conditions and terms of receiving payment for services, and for a long time, particularly with the aid of various scientific and quasi-scientific terms utilized as standards for communication, and created and sustained an aura of protection and immunity against outside scrutiny. Under these circumstances at least initially it was very difficult for nonphysicians to assess the true impact outside interference had (by governments, third-party payers, etc.) on the quality of care. This hegemony continued to prevail for many decades, but, ironically, appears to have set its own limits if not demise. The process simply attracted too much of society's interests and concern. The emerging high healthcare costs, in particular the excessive annual rates of growth in healthcare costs which far outpaced the rate of inflation for other items in the Consumer Price Index basket of goods and services attracted attention sufficient if not more than sufficient for prompting closer social and legal scrutiny of the inner workings of the medical profession.

Policies and programs designed to combat costs and overutilization of healthcare services gave rise to concerns that efforts aimed at meeting cost control targets will miss quality control targets. That is, costs will be controlled, or at least attempts in that direction will be made at the expense of quality. Trade-offs between cost control and quality control were perceived to be inevitable by many. Congress' concern for healthcare quality within the Medicare program may be noted from the very early stages of the Program started in 1965. The Experimental Medical Care Review Organizations, and the subsequent Professional Standards Review Organizations (PSROs) in the early 1970s were aimed at ensuring some minimum professional standards in healthcare delivery to Medicare beneficiaries. In 1982, the creation of the Utilization and Quality Control Peer Review Organizations ("PROs") further evidenced federal concerns with healthcare quality for Medicare beneficiaries. Yet, problems inherent in the definition of healthcare quality persisted.

Efforts to define health itself perennially suffer from various problems, as I mentioned in the previous chapter. One problem is the diversity of dimensions that go into the concept of health, the differences among these dimensions from patient to patient, various notions of attainability regarding health, and, perhaps most importantly, the often obscured relationship between various health services (care processes - which themselves are often difficult to discern), and the result (outcome) which again is a multidimensional notion with various interpretations for various persons, can be a convergence of various physical, psychological, spiritual and personal dimensions: it may often happen that good process is followed by favorable outcome, while service of questionable quality can also be accompanied by acceptable results. Thus, if care quality is not precisely linked, or linkable, to service then how can provider accountability be implemented? These problems are integral parts of efforts to define care quality.

Definition Efforts by the National Academy of Sciences

In early 1974, the Institute of Medicine (Institute), of the National Academy of Sciences, advanced the following statement regarding healthcare quality assurance:

"The primary goal of quality assurance system should be to make health care effective in bettering the health status and satisfaction of a population, within the resources which society and individuals have chosen to spend for that care"1.

While this statement emphasizes the importance of economic constraints, it does not provide a definition of quality. Subsequently, the Institute collected some 100 definitions of healthcare quality from the literature from which it synthesized the following definition:

"quality of care is the degree to which health services for individuals and populations increase the likelihood of desired health outcomes and are consistent with current professional knowledge"2.

Here we may note a reference to a yardstick ("degree"). It attempts to be comprehensive ("health services") and target oriented by noting an outcome ("desired health outcome"). By referring to "likelihood" it allows for chance outcomes that may often prevail pursuant to any care, and notes the relationship between care and outcome. Finally, the definition relates health service quality to accepted and current professional standards, thus giving expression to the need for state of the technical competence. It may be noted that the Institute omitted references to economic resource constraints or availability either at the personal or social levels, in order not to dilute the definition, measurement and concern for care quality with factors otherwise not healthcare in nature. This omission appears to disregard one of the two main policy issues involved in the healthcare reform debate of 1994, namely cost containment. Although it is understood that cost containment efforts may in some instances compromise quality, these efforts are not envisioned for implementation with the understanding that they should, or even could very well, compromise quality. Thus, what we perhaps should consider is a bilateral constraint relationship: optimum quality subject to cost constraints, and costs ceilings (efficiency) subject to a minimum socially and individually acceptable quality standard. Furthermore, individually and socially acceptable standards may also be considered. While adequate or better healthcare maybe produced for some or most individuals, they cannot be for society as a whole without the reallocation resources from their alternative applications, thus causing additional dilemmas and decision needs as to which alternative resource application is more desirable, and to what degree, generating problems with virtually unresolvable social and political implications.

The need for healthcare is acquired, in most instances, involuntarily. Its administration can have life-death consequences. Thus, the healthcare product is seen as being quite different from other products. Its contents include not only hopefully measurable dimensions of a technical nature but also highly subjective elements such as patient-provider trust and affinity, and various other notions of psychological comfort, in an era of proliferating malpractice litigation, for both sides of the transaction. This complex relationship is made even more difficult by conflicts between the provider's economic interests and the welfare of the patient, conflicts which have been introduced by various pre-paid and fee-for-service payments systems, as well as by third-party payers such as Medicare and Medicaid, where efforts to control costs are often difficult to reconcile with possibly opposing efforts to control quality, particularly when both of these efforts emanate from the same source.

The Institute's definition of healthcare quality was a culmination of many elements from a large number of definitions surveyed from the relevant literature. Some key elements were discerned from these definitions. Thus, some sort of *ranking* of provider service above the minimum acceptable level is needed in order to distinguish by some standard merely acceptable service from that which is outstanding. Terms such as "degree", "level", "highest", and other similar ones imply some level of service built into definitions. Because of the varied terminology used in the literature, another element needs to *identify* what is being defined, "healthcare", "medical care", "patient care", in terms of provider performance, care actually received (or perceived to have been received) by the patient, or by segments of society.

A related element in need of identification, especially in definitions emphasizing outcome (instead of structure and process - all discussed earlier in the volume) is the *target entity* of care. Is it a patient, a customer, an HMO member, a Medicare or Medicaid beneficiary, or entire segments of society, or of a subset of society? The variety of terms used almost matches the variety of definitions surveyed.

The *goals* of the care is clearly an important and frequently included element in a definition. Thus, the ability to coordinate structure and process to secure some desired outcome may be a valid goal. In fact, the relationship may be bilateral, as not only the interaction between structure and process that will impact on outcome, but some predetermined outcome may contribute to the determination of what structure and process would be most desirable. Furthermore, healthcare goals may be developer specific, that is, they differ with the developer of the quality definition: third-party payers, hospital administrators, individual providers, government agencies, may each see a different goal paramount enough to be included in a definition of healthcare quality. In addition, goals such as patient satisfaction and perceived outcomes may be as important as medically technical goals such as the biomedical outcome of the care. The problem with the latter may be that a patient does not have the necessary quality or quantity of information or data to actually form an educated opinion, and while satisfaction may be of some significance, or even highly significant, at the termination of care, that satisfaction may in fact be superficial if symptoms or results of inadequate care are delayed substantially. In other words, goals in quality definitions need somehow to be time-stamped so as to allow adequate time period for properly discerning the results of care, and *all* results of that care.

All healthcare processes carry some elements of *risks*, such as side-effects, or less than expected or even unexpected outcomes. Thus, some predictions are needed as elements of quality definition, predictions regarding risks and benefits, and the probability of their occurrence. However, serious complexities in this regard need to be dealt with which may make the formulation of a broadly or uniformly applicable care quality definition difficult: risks and benefits may be individual patient or procedure specific with considerable degrees of variation in both respects. This element was considered in a definition formulated by the JCAHO, where healthcare quality was seen as "The degree to which patient care services increase the probability of desired patient outcomes and reduce the probability of undesired outcomes, given the current state of knowledge"[3].

Another important element of a care quality definition need to reflect on what *specific outcome* is expected from a care quality of some level. What specific benefits (dimensions of health) should be expected to accrue from the care? More general benefits attributed to care of individuals might be stated such as "independent existence", "level of well-being", "level of well-being" or attained "clinical well-being", while more specific ones likely attributed to broader patient groups or social segments may refer to outcomes in terms of lower morbidity and mortality levels in the population, social and psychological well-being, or results that sustain or restore functioning. Once again, these elements of care definition may be inadequate, even misleading, unless appropriate time dimensions are added. Much of the outcome may depend on the information provided to the provider by the patient, the extent to which the patient follows provider advice, and other similar *participatory elements* that need to be attributed to the patient.

Technical *competence* of the provider, and provider performance that may be constrained by the *existing state* of technology and scientific knowledge need to be fundamental elements of any care quality definition. Competence itself is a broad concept that goes beyond scientific knowledge. It must also take into consideration perceptual, manual, and cognitive as well as management skills, with the latter becoming more important with the increasing emergence of medical practice in corporate and organizational settings, and it must also consider the extent of primary dedication and loyalty to the patients in contrast to economically or leisure motivated self-interests. Important balance is added to the definition by allowing for constraints upon the implementation of all dimensions of technical competence, constraints such as limits on achievable levels of quality due insufficient knowledge, limited technology, and the current state of scientific knowledge. Since the state of medical knowledge and technology is highly dynamic and constantly changing, and in some areas even in a state flux with frequently occurring contradicting changes, care quality definitions also need to be adjusted to accommodate these changes. Thus, any complete definition of healthcare quality should be viewed as a dynamic process, instead of a static one.

An important element imbedded in human nature and relationships is the *interpersonal skills* of the provider: mutual trust, dealing with patient concerns at the time the service is rendered and on a continuing basis. If one assumes that patient psychology in relation to an actual or perceived malady is an important determinant of outcome on a dynamic basis, then the effective exercise of interpersonal skills on the part of the physician may be viewed as an important process or even structural element in the global context of care quality.

Another element of quality definition may relate to existing *practice standards*. In other words, quality is noted in the light of a comparison between service performed (in some structural context) along with some expected outcome and some professionally or legally recognized and accepted standards. Levels of poor quality would reflect downward deviations from those standards. Acceptable quality would simply be at the standard level, and levels of excellence would somehow be characterized by upward deviations from the standard. Unless quantified, the comparison process may hide various hidden pitfalls and excessive subjectivities which may be difficult to deal with. Thus, quantification of the standards and of the objects of comparison need to be accomplished, a matter which will be looked at later on in this chapter.

Finally, and by no means to the exclusion of additional elements that may enter into a healthcare quality definition, *resource constraints* may be an important element, although we have seen that the Institute has not alluded to it in its definition cited here earlier. An important consideration in this context is whether varying resource constraints may need to or should give rise to varying rigors for care quality definitions, a consideration which would add substantial additional, perhaps socially unjustified, complexities to an already convoluted maze of issues involved in the task. Are we to imply that whatever standard definition criteria are accepted for a given socio-economic level of society, that it be compromised for those with more stringent resource constraints but enhanced for those with a more generous endowment of resources? For if we did, it may not in fact be much of a deviation from real life circumstances where the quality of healthcare (however defined) provided within specific ranges above mortality may in most cases depend upon the expected financial returns to the provider which, in turn, often reflect, directly or indirectly, upon the financial resources of the patient. However, to generate various levels of care quality definitions for social consumption that reflect on these inequalities is likely to be politically prohibitive. Alternatively, one socially acceptable care quality definition could be generated for society as a whole, reflecting on economic constraints, and, at least theoretically, averaging out various care level possibilities may refer to some optimum levels of care, rather than to the ultimately best or ideal levels of care which may in some selected cases also be attainable. Thus, some theoretical optimum rather than ideal level of care may be provided with the available amount of resources under the assumption that those resources are used in a most efficient manner. However, one must also note that the latter caveat, namely efficiency in medicine and in the various phases of medical care, is in itself an almost unmanageably complex issue. Furthermore, how can one reconcile this optimum level of care with that which providers may consider absolutely necessary in the face of specific medical problems is another matter to contend with. Finally, in what proportion or ratio are resource constraints to be allocated, if at all, among the process, structure and outcome dimensions of health care quality definitions, particularly in view of the complex multilateral relationships among these dimensions, as we discussed them earlier[4].

Rational Consumer Behavior and Healthcare Service Choices[5]

If we assume people's neutrality towards gambles, choices under uncertainty may be predicted by using the expected utility theory (EUT) method. Although developed to predict choice alternatives among financial outcomes, EUT can also be used to analyze risky clinical decision choice alternatives among health outcomes, that is, comparing choices among a number of medical treatments and their potential outcomes. The risk may be associated with the uncertain outcomes of given medical treatments where each medical treatment can be viewed as a risky option, where associated with each such option is a set of possible outcomes along with their probabilities.

Expected utility theory of risky choice behavior may be illustrated as follows, using gambling events. A person can have two choices, gamble or not gamble. If he chooses not to gamble he wins nothing and loses nothing. His utility is $U(0)$. If he gambles, he receives a price **w** with a probability **p** or he loses **v** with an attached probability of **(1–p)**. Whether or not the person decides to gamble depends on his attitude to gambling, which may be neutral, risk averter, or risk lover. If his gambling utility is *neutral*, his expected utility is $EU = pU(w) + (1–p)U(v) = U[pw + (1–p)v]$, $U(w)$ and $U(v)$ being the utilities associated with the prize and loss receptively. The equality is brought about by the assumption of neutrality. Thus, if $pw + (1–p)v$, i.e. the expected winning, is > or = zero, then he will choose to gamble since not gambling yields him the utility of $U(0)$, and his utility function will be increasing. In cases of *risk aversion*, the expected utility is $EU = pU(w) + [(1–p)U(v)]$, which is < than $U[pw + (1–p)v]$]. This means that the person prefers to get the expected value of the gamble, $pw + (1–p)v$, rather than gamble. Since $pU(w) + (1–p)U(v) < U[pw + (1–p)v]$, the choice will be not to gamble even if the expected value (winnings) from the gamble $pw + (1–p)v$ is > 0. Risk aversions are typically depicted by concave functions, and are normally assumed in the expected utility theory. Finally, *risk loving* situations are depicted by functions inverse to risk aversion. The person prefers gambling itself to the expected value of the gamble. Even if the expected value (winning) from a gamble is < 0, he may choose to gamble because his expected utility $EU = pU(w) + (1–p)U(v)$ may be > than $U[pw + (1–p)v]$. Risk loving situations are reflected by convex functions.

A number of studies have found that people do not always choose between risky options according to the standards of expected utility theory[6], nor is EUT found to be able to predict demand for health insurance based on risky choices[7]. Models involving risky options associated with alternative monetary outcomes also indicate that people are often not gambling neutrals favoring some outcomes to highly probable ones.

A study of lung cancer patients choice of one treatment over another was based almost entirely on expected survival, suggesting risk neutrality since the utility of the gamble itself is equal to the utility of the expected value of (winnings from) the gamble[8]. This means that if expected survival time of treatment **A** exceeds the survival period brought about by **B**, then the utility of **A** > than utility of **B**. So, the selection of the treatment with the longest expected survival is an optimal selection only if the patient is risk neutral. Risk neutrality in this context then may be defined as [1] $U(G) = U(p_1X_1 + p_2X_2)$, with $U(G) =$ the utility of gamble with p_1 chance of X_1 years of survival and p_2 chance of X_2 years of survival, and holds if a person is indifferent towards gambles involving years of life and values each year of expected life equally. Equation [1] can further restate gambling neutrality as [2] $U(G) = p_1U(X_1) + p_2U(X_2)$, and give rise to a linear utility of life years function, if the person also values each future year of life equally, such as $U(X_i) = aX_i$, where **a** is a constant, so that [3] $p_1U(x_1) + p_2U(X_2) = p_1aX_1 + p_2aX_2 = a(p_1X_1 + p_2X_2) = p_1X_1 + p_2X_2)$, satisfying equation [2], and the choice of treatment on the basis of expected survival assumes patient neutrality towards the gamble attaching equal value to each year of expected life.

In arriving at a rational decision whether or not to treat operable lung cancer with surgery, the lung cancer study derived a utility function of expected life years by using so called *certainty equivalents* (CE). Within the context of risk and uncertainty, variable values assume at least two characteristics, an average (mean) value, and a yardstick measuring the riskiness or uncertainty surrounding that average, such as a standard deviation. A CE procedure entails a value determination for a variable such that the individual is indifferent between that value, which is assumed as attainable with certainty, and some higher mean (gamble) value of the variable but with a standard deviation equal to zero. Lung cancer patients were to choose indifference between some fixed period (i.e. the CE between the gamble and immediate death) of certain survival and a 50:50 chance of surviving for 25 years and immediate death. That is, the patients attain 50% of the 25 years survival utility during the fixed period of certain survival, or they attain a 25% of the 25 year survival utility by getting the CE for a 50:50 gamble between the first CE and immediate death. In this fashion a utility function can be generated for the patients, provided they are neutral toward gambles and as to each year of life, i.e. [4] U_{50} = .5U(25) + .5U(0) = .5U(25) or equal to the utility of a gamble with a 50% chance of 25 years of survival and a 50% chance of death.

Another survey was conducted involving some 50 employees, of both genders, of the US Government between ages 25 and 50 (the results, incidentally, were found to be gender and age neutral). The survey centered on two questions: (a) assuming good health throughout, did they value each of the next 30 years of life equally, and (b) addressed the risk posture of the participants by calculating the CE of a 50:50 gamble between death and 30 years of life. People are risk neutral with respect to years of life when they value each year of life equally and are neutral towards gambles. Thus, if people value each year of life equally and are risk averse are not neutral towards gambles and do not behave in accordance with the EUT, and nor do those who value years in the distant future more than years in the near future, are risk averse and are not neutral towards gambles. Of the 50 people surveyed, 19 indicated that they valued each year of life equally, and 18 of this 19 selected CEs under 15 years suggesting risk aversity with respect to years of life, and aversity to gambles. The other 31 indicated that they did not value each year of life equally and selected CEs less than 15 years suggesting risk aversity

Additional findings suggested that there is significant variability in the risk attitudes among individuals for any given gamble, and there is also significant variability in the risk attitudes of given individuals toward different gambles. The variability of a given individual to different gambles suggests that risk attitudes are not absolute but are a function of the parameters in the gamble, and that people generally become more risk averse as the probability of death in a gamble increases.

Social and Policy Implications of Healthcare Quality

There are a number of issues which, while not inherent in the definition of healthcare quality itself, are closely related to it either causally or consequentially. Firstly, issues such as healthcare expenditures, third-party payment systems and practices such as those by Medicare, Medicaid, and managed care organizations are all very important. Secondly, directly payment related issues such as utilization management and reviews, alteration of care environment from inpatient to ambulatory settings, and access to care, also need to be looked at when examining healthcare quality related issues. Thirdly, the broad areas of healthcare quality assurance (a subject to be examined in depth later in the volume) such as professional accountability and responsibility, malpractice and risk management are also of clear concern. Finally, issues imbedded in various healthcare regulatory statutes and public perceptions of healthcare as being virtually a "public good", all have direct relevance to discussions on, and definitions of, healthcare quality.

In 1993, the US spent over $800 million on healthcare, amounting to over 14% of the GNP. About 75% of this went for financing health services and supplies, the rest for capital expenditures, facilities and research[9]. These expenditures follow a consistent average annual rate of growth which far exceeds that in other sectors of the US economy. Thus, between 1970 and 1990, national income absorbed by healthcare increased by over 50% (from 7.3% of GNP in 1970 to 12.3% in 1990), and may be projected to reach about 16% by the year 2000. Yet, the number of people without health insurance increased from about 30 million in 1979 to over 37 million in 1987. These may be viewed in the backdrop of 1965 when national healthcare expenditures were at a relatively low level of about $42 billion, some 6% of the US GNP[10]. Similar increases were registered for Medicare expenditures which amount just over $7 billion in 1970 but were at $35 billion in 1980, about $82 billion in 1987, and more than $130 billion in 1993.

In the past, various forms of price controls and *cost containment* efforts were implemented, such as Medicare's Prospective Payment System [PPS] with thus far unascertained impact on the quality of care. It has been noted, however, that PPS has shortened hospital stays, the average length of stay (ALOS), with an increasing flow of inpatients deemed to be releasable from the hospital environment into more ambulatory or home care (less expensive) environments to complete recovery. Questions have been raised, without confirmed answers, whether unduly early release of patients from hospitals may have, or are, contributing the a decrease in the quality of care[11]. The matter is further complicated by the various social, political and ethical considerations which conflict with economic ones. Poverty, homelessness, substance abuse and other factors which themselves generate poor health and the consequent need for additional healthcare expenditures continue to proliferate. In addition, the perennial federal budget deficit, and frequent local government deficits, which take occasional but certainly recurring political heat often overshadow other political, social and ethical considerations, such as providing insurance coverage to some 37 million people who are without that coverage in a typical year.

The financial predicament in which *physicians* find themselves due to various fee payment and financial incentive systems may also inhibit care quality. Many providers are unhappy with the Medicare physician payment system[12], notwithstanding the fact healthcare expenditures directed at physicians have consistently increased over the years. Many physicians still refuse to accept Medicare assignments, and often charge additional out-of-pocket fees to their patients, when the latter may also have to contend with copayments imposed upon them by insurance carriers. Patients restrained by financial exigencies may need to reconsider accessing medical care, even if the latter is accessible, and if they do and the latter is, it may likely be of the quality substantially less than standard.

In order to improve efficiency and effectiveness in care delivery, that is, to assure at least standard care is delivered when necessary, in quantities deemed necessary to all who need it, where they need it (i.e. inpatient or ambulatory) in a timely fashion, while controlling costs at the same time, elaborate care *utilization management* programs have been implemented in healthcare delivery settings, in particular with those delivered by managed care organizations functioning in the private sector. Care quality may be compromised if utilization controls and limits are excessively, discriminately or unduly implemented, thus limiting or precluding necessary care[13]. This may be the case notwithstanding carefully implemented quality assurance programs, where the latter may come into real conflict with various utilization management and utilization review efforts, particularly by third-party payers. Following practice guidelines which in major institutions have become important policy ingredients may mitigate this conflict[14].

The evolution of fierce price *competition* for patients in the market place among providers and among insurers, as evidenced by advertising and other marketing campaigns of increasing intensity, the relentless push for increases in market shares on the part of institutions within any relevant geographic markets, could cause medical care to become less personal. Care may become merely a commodity which is to be produced and delivered at a minimum cost, subject to competition and third-party payer determined price constraints, where unless carefully monitored quality may become a cushion to make-up for lost profitability. These trends may be accelerated by the growth of for-profit investor owned healthcare providing institutions, and also by the increasing integration between the financing and delivery functions of healthcare. The latter phenomena place the provider at a financial risk through the implementation of various cost conscious payment systems, such as the Medicare prospective payments system, and various forms of capitated fee structures.

In the previous chapter we looked at the many dimensions involved in the delivery of total healthcare. The process in general is multidimensional in terms of the stages involved, and the people participating at each stage of the delivery. Each stage and each contributor at each stage has had their impact on the process and the ultimate outcome, if in fact the ultimate outcome (other than mortality) can be clearly timed and identified. All of these, identifiable to various extents, elements have an impact on the quality of care provided. Thus, if quality is compromised, the source of the compromise may need to be traced back to any one or more of these contributing elements for purposes of attaching responsibility and accountability. The process is further complicated by the fact that the patient's preferences, needs, and treatment responses tend to vary. Different outcomes may be generated by different provider groups and different processes for the same patient, and the same provider group with the same process may generate different outcomes with different patients. The distinction between caused and chance outcomes becomes confusing at best. The point of clear responsibility for a malfeasance may become difficult to identify, even if that malfeasance can be causally isolated from a possible series malfeasances committed independently, or as a result of an original malfeasance occurred earlier in the process. In other words, infringement(s) on care quality can occur independently from one another, or can be causally interrelated by earlier infringements causing an undesired alteration in the care process in later stages, each having their negative impact on outcome.

The attempted assignment of responsibility under this is what may be called an *accountability web*. While clearly difficult, it may be achieved in two categories of actions, private and public, often without clear lines of separation. In the private category, the direct provider's sense of professional responsibility manifested in terms of codes of ethics, or by way of an implied contract (or fiduciary responsibility) between the provider and his patients whereby the provider commits competence and integrity, has typically been in the past considered to be the basis for reliance[15]. However, with the increased emergence of market based competition among providers, the proliferation of medical malpractice litigation directed against individual and institutional providers (notwithstanding the fact that no more than about 10% of actual medical malfeasances end up in litigation) this traditional perception of professionalism as a basis for quality self-control must have lost considerable credibility. Yet, the willingness on the part of hospitals to voluntarily participate in external evaluations and accreditation processes, such as those implemented by the JCAHO, and the internal implementation of various types of quality assurance programs, even if prompted by pervasive risk management control to avoid legal malpractice exposure, indicates that self-imposed professional standards are still a viable means for care quality control.

Healthcare quality is not only a concern to the individual but also to society, in fact, social healthcare status may often be a source of negative or positive externalities for individuals, and vice versa. Because of this, governments have taken on some of the responsibilities for at least attempting to monitor healthcare quality. In order to secure, although only indirectly with minimum standards for quality, government agencies have long been licensing healthcare professionals and certifying institutions. In addition, health planning programs, certificate of need requirements, utilization and cost controls, and compulsory quality assurance programs have long been implemented in government financed healthcare delivery systems. Federal assistance of residency training programs and the National Health Service Corporation were designed to improve access to and the distribution of providers. It should be noted, however, that as far as care quality improvement efforts are concerned, recent years have seen the assimilation of HCFA mandated quality assurance programs designed for Medicare patients into the general competitively motivated marketing efforts by hospitals to gain market shares in all patient areas not just those with Medicare coverage.

The government's involvement in the distribution and limited monitoring of healthcare delivery may be attributed to the perception of healthcare services as public goods, or at the least, a set of responsibilities that belong to the public. Within the context of economics, a "public good" (service) is one that is consumed collectively with a utility for society as a whole, and where one person cannot prevent another person from consuming it by imposing a price or cost. A public good's consumption cannot be rivaled by another person and its consumption by one person does not alter its availability to others[16]. Thus, it has frequently been advocated that all members of society should be availed some "adequate" level of care ("adequate" rarely · defined - adequately)[17]. To assure access at reasonable cost, or financed for the poor most efficiently by way allocated public funds, the private market system may not be relied on for investment in data research and information dissemination as expected returns may not warrant such expenditures. Enters the public sector, with information collected, processed and distributed to the population at large. The "public" nature of healthcare may also be interpreted therefore as one where the health of individuals, at least their freedom from many types of highly contagious or infectious diseases benefits society as a whole by ridding it of the dangers of spreading.

Notes

1. National Academy of Sciences, Institute of Medicine, *Advancing the Quality of Health Care*, A Policy Statement by a Committee of the Institute of Medicine, Washington, DC, 1974.
2. Lohr, K. (ed), *Medicare: A Strategy for Quality Assurance*, National Academy of Sciences, Committee of the Institute of Medicine, Vol. I, Washington, DC, p. 21.
3. Joint Commission on Accreditation of Healthcare Organizations 1990, *Accreditation Manual for Hospitals*, Chicago, IL, 1989.
4. Lohr, K. (ed), *Medicare: A Strategy for Quality Assurance*, Vol. II, National Academy Press, Washington, DC, 1990, Ch. 5. For a review of some of the definitions cited, see Brook, R.H., Kosecoff, J.B., "Commentary, Competition and Quality", *Health Affairs,* Vol. 7, Summer 1988; Steffen, G.E., "Quality of Medical Care: A Definition", *JAMA*, Vol. 260, 1988; Lee, R.I. and Jones, W.L., *The Fundamentals of Good Medical Care*, University of Chicago Press, Chicago, IL, 1933; Sanazaro, P.J., Worth, R.M., "Concurrent Quality Assurance in Hospital Care", New England Journal of Medicine, Vol. 298, 1978; Donabedian, A., *Explorations in Quality Assessment and Monitoring, Vol. I. The Definition of Quality and Approaches to its Assessment,* Health Administration Press, Ann Arbor, MI, 1980; Lohr, K.N. and Brook, R.H., *Quality Assurance in Medicine: Experience in the Public Sector*, R-3139-HHS, The Rand Corporation, Santa Monica, CA, 1984.
5. This section relies on Hellinger, F.J., "Expected Utility Theory and Risky Choices with Health Outcomes", *Medical Care,* Vol. 27, No. 3, March 1989. For a systematic discussion on the economics of uncertainty, the reader is also referred to Denton, A., *Economics and Consumer Behavior,* Cambridge University Press, 1980, Ch. 14; and Varian, H., *Microeconomic Analysis*, W.W. Norton, New York, 1992, Ch. 11.
6. These were cited by Hellinger: Machina, M.J., "Choice Under Uncertainty: Problems Solved and Unsolved", *The Journal of Economic Perspectives*, Vol. 1, 1987. Shoemaker, P.J.H., "The Expected Utility Model: Its Variants, Purposes, Evidence and Limitations", *Journal of Economic Literature*, Vol. 20, 1982. Slovic, P., Lichtenstein, S., "Preference Reversals: A Broader Perspective", *American Economic Review*, Vol. 73, 1985. Heiner, R.A., "Origin of Predictable Behavior: Further Modeling and Applications", *American Economic Review*, Vol. 75, 1985.
7. Marquis, M.S., Holmer, M.R., *Choice Under Uncertainty and the Demand for Health Insurance*, Rand Corporation, Santa Monica, CA, December 1986.
8. McNeil, B.J., Weichselbaum, R., Pauker, S., "Fallacy of the Five Year Survival in Lung Cancer", *New England Journal of Medicine,* Vol. 299, 1978.
9. Seplaki, L., *Cost and Competition in American Medicine: Theory, Policy and Institutions*, University Press of America, Lanham, MD, 1994, Ch. 11.
10. Seplaki, L., 1994, Ch. 27.
11. Kahn, K.L., Rubenstein, L.V., Kosecoff, J., "DRG-Based Prospective Payment System and Quality of Care", *AFCR Clinical Epidemiology and Health Care,*

Clinical Research, Vol. 37, No. 2, 1989. See also Fitzgerald, J.F., Moore, P.S., Dittus, R.S., "The Care of Elderly Patients with Hip Fracture", *New England Journal of Medicine,* Vol. 319, 1988, and Fitzgerald, J.F., Fagan, L.F., Tierney, W.M. et al., "Changing Patterns of Hip Fracture Care Before and After Implementation of the Prospective Payment System", *JAMA,* Vol. 258, 1987. Prospective Payment Assessment Commission, *Medical Prospective Payment and the American Healthcare System, Report to Congress,* Washington, DC, 1989, and also by PROPAC, *Medical Prospective Payment and the American Healthcare System, Report to Congress,* Washington, DC, 1988.

12.   Physician Payment Review Commission, *Annual Report*(s) *to Congress,* Washington, DC, 1988, 1989, 1990.

13.   We will take a close look at the impact of HMOs and other managed care organizations on healthcare quality later in the volume.

14.   Utilization management and review issues in this context are discussed in Gray, B.H. and Field, M.J. (eds), *Controlling Costs and Changing Patient Care? The Role of Utilization Management,* National Academy Press, Washington, DC, 1989, and Brown, R.E., Sheingold, S.H. and Luce, B.R., *Options for Using Practice Guidelines in Reducing the Volume of Medically Unnecessary Services,* BHARC-013/89/027. Battelle Human Affairs Research Center, Washington, DC, June 1989.

15.   Pellegrino, E.D., "A Humanistic Base for Professional Ethics in Medicine", *New York State Journal of Medicine,* Vol. 77, August 1977; Vladeck, B.C., "Quality Assurance Through External Control", *Inquiry,* Vol. 25, 1988; Farber, S.J., "Perspectives in Quality Assurance and Technology" in *Quality of Care and Technology Assessment,* National Academy Press, Washington, DC, 1988.

16.   A "private good" may be consumed exclusively by the purchaser and others may have no legal access to it without the consent of the owner. Thus, one person's consumption of a private good precludes another person from consuming the same unit. Total demand for a private good is generated by a simple horizontal addition of individual demand curves for that good [refer to any basic microeconomic text]. The total demand curve for a public good is obtained by a vertical addition of the individual demand curves.

17.   Goldsmith, J.C., "Commentary: Competition's Impact: A Report From the Front", *Health Affairs,* Vol. 7, Summer 1988. Leader, S., Moon, M. (ed), "Forging the Agenda" in *Changing America's Healthcare System,* Scott Forsman & Company, Glenview, IL, 1989. Arnold, M.D., "The Politics of Ensuring Quality of Care for Elders", *Generation,* Vol. 13, Winter 1989. Enthoven, A., "Managed Competition: An Agenda for Action", *Health Affairs,* Vol. 7, Summer 1988.

4 Measuring Healthcare Quality: Broad Issues

Healthcare quality is a matter not only for society's well-being and the well-being of its members, i.e. the patients, but it has also become a significant consideration in the financial markets. In the context of credit worthiness of a hospital and for investors in general, quality and financial performance factors are closely related. Lacking better measurable quality indices at the present, factors such as hospital market shares, physician loyalty, board certification, and malpractice track record are proxies often used by external evaluators of hospital financial strength. Government generated hospital-specific mortality statistics are normally considered unacceptable by themselves, unless serious adjustments are made for patient risk and patient-mix factors. Market shares and their historical trends in particular, are considered a useful proxy at this time, since it is assumed that people with adequate information will gravitate to providers with the lowest cost and the best quality performance. Thus, society's interest in healthcare quality goes beyond the ethical and welfare issues related to the various dimension of quality discussed earlier. It is also imbedded in the financial health of the healthcare industry and in the returns that industry provides to its investors. With the increase in the proportion of investor owned institutional providers, in contrast to those which have traditionally provided service on a not-for profit basis, these considerations have become more important in recent years. Furthermore, it can also be argued that the precise causal relationship between healthcare quality and financial performance of providers may be a circuitous one: better quality healthcare will attract larger numbers of patients and will increase market share which, with controlled costs, increase the profitability and investment perceived performance of the provider. This, in turn, may financially enable the provider to procure better facilities and other ingredients (such as more competent personnel and better monitoring facilities) normally associated with healthcare service *structures* yielding a more reliable *process* and better *outcome*, using the traditional hierarchies for healthcare quality definitions and measurements. This would in some way

relate healthcare quality to size, and the latter to better financial performance, back to size, and perhaps quality. In order to facilitate the understanding of the nature and magnitude of these relationships, *quality* in healthcare
itself needs to be understood. The previous chapter dealt with some definitional issues. In this chapter, we will examine some measurement and
measurement related issues.

One of the underlying queries may address the entity or entities that
would be called upon in the first place to measure or assess the quality of
healthcare. One alternative solution to the dilemma is to have the *patient* do
the assessment[1]. After all if the consumer has a sufficient amount of relevant
and correct information, and if he/she possesses the necessary competence to
evaluate that information, he/she should be able to assess the quality of
healthcare service received. Based on neoclassical price theory, one could
add further that as healthcare market competition increases, the prices of
healthcare services will approach their true cost, and consumers, equipped
with the necessary amount and quality of information can decide for themselves what to buy and where to buy it.

However, this sounds like, and may in fact be not more than, *healthcare market utopia*. One main problem area is the quantity and quality of
information available to the patient and the patient's ability to process or
utilize that information for evaluation or assessment purposes. There are
various degrees of patient ignorance factors in this area, factors which
depend on the nature of the information needed, that is, the technical complexity of the data and information necessary to understand the process
involved and their possible outcomes for the patient, and upon the patient's
sophistication and even basic educational background as well as attitude
needed to meaningfully asses any information. Some patients blindly trust
their physicians, for better or worse. In other situations, the provider may for
whatever reasons and under whatever circumstances not be in the position or
not wish to divulge all the necessary or pertinent information to the patient.
In extreme cases where the patient is unconscious or incompetent for any
other reasons, choice by the patient based on information, even if the latter is
perfect and timely, is not a likely possibility; although one could argue that
such choice in some cases may be made even then by the patient's family or
other legal representative, provided there is time to exercise such judgment.
In other words, and notwithstanding the staunchest information advocates, it
is unlikely that a patient or his/her representative will spend time shopping
around for quality and price with the presence of obvious and severe heart

attack symptoms - normally the geographically closest institution is chosen, at least for the initial stages of care.

The situation is further complicated by the increasingly emerging role of individual providers as "healthcare double-agents": namely, that for the patient wherein the providers provide advice, information, and recommendation to the patient and even procures services on behalf of the patient, and that for other interest groups, particularly in managed care environments, who may be motivated more by financial considerations than the patient's welfare, or may be motivated by the patient's welfare where such motivations may be obscured by stringent financial constraints. Under these circumstances of double-agency, two possibly irreconcilable sets of performance evaluations may be called for or may come forth, one from the patients and the other from the provider's employer(s) or third-party payers.

Another alternative as to who should evaluate provider performance, one that appears to have been implemented for some time in various forms, is *peer groups*, and professional organizations. We have discussed these processes in the previous chapters. It should be noted though that to the extent that these professional evaluations tend to judge providers at or immediately past the educational stage, such as the contents and minimum standards for training, examinations and accreditations, credentialing and licensing, they do not judge the quality of performance in the process of care delivery. Although it can be argued that the higher the quality requirements at these performance-preliminary stages, the better the actual care delivery performance will be at later stages, allowing for reasonable time factors.

A third, and perhaps an inevitable alternative performance evaluator may be various *governments* and the third-party payers themselves. These entities spend moneys on healthcare on behalf of their insured, enrolled members, or statutory beneficiaries. Claims for such moneys are inherently competing for scarce resources, and the payers' social as well as private responsibility to ascertain the nature of delivered services has been becoming a *de facto* accepted matter. Once again, these entities may evaluate care and define accepted standards and delivered care differently from those of patients or provider groups.

Once the entities for performing healthcare quality measurements are in place, numerous tasks, even in broad terms as discussed here, need to be dealt with. In particular, the dimension(s) of quality to be measured needs to be determined. If we are to measure quality in terms of *outcome*, then the service generated improvement in health status needs to be determined, and the services applied need to be compared with alternative services with their possible outcomes, along with the likelihoods attached to those outcomes, as well as the comparative costs involved. In some cases, it may be difficult to ascertain let alone compare outcomes for different service alternatives. For instance, if a nurse looks in on a patient four times per day versus six times per day, with no particular noted change in the patient's health status how can outcome differential be measured?, i.e. whether and to what extent the patient has benefited, beyond simply implying that the more (higher frequency) nursing attention a patient gets the better his or her health status likely to evolve (other things, of course, held constant).

Notwithstanding outcome determination related problems of this type of situation, the *process* aspects can easily be compared. Assuming other factors constant, from any one patient's point of view, the more visits the better. There are no direct and obvious measurability problems. But that may not always be the case. What about consistently differing practice styles among physicians? How does one measure practice styles and interpersonal relationships? To measure quality under these circumstances, *structural* variables are most likely to come to the, rather tenuous, rescue. Thus, factors such as appointment schedules, physical facilities, capital, diagnostic and therapeutic facilities, and the size of the medical and allied medical support staff need to be examined as alternatives to outright process measurements.

Professional accountability needs another look. With institutionally employed providers, accountability is implemented within the institutional hierarchies along lines of staff seniority. Self-employed practitioners see accountability as an interference with professional autonomy. So, while they accept peer review procedures, accountability is still a threatening notion to most providers. Yet the trend towards increased and intensified accountability, in fact multilateral accountability, has become evident during the past decade or so. Healthcare cost acceleration and social as well as political issues that arose as a result mandate a ranking of priorities. Third-party payers, private and public (governments), self-insured and externally insured employers, all need to make decisions regarding how much to spend in healthcare and importantly for what. The task is to determine medical practices that generate desired outcomes for the largest segments of the population in the most efficient and cost effective manner. The complexities of the measurement and definitional processes and issues involved, as already discussed to an extent in the volume, may make this statement of task no more than an exercise in healthcare quality measurement utopia, however, the need is real and the problems have to be dealt with as much as possible.

It may be that the trend towards increasingly involving the healthcare service consumer, i.e. increasing provider accountability to their patients, possesses a good part of the answer. A later chapter in this volume will examine the intricacies involved in this process. However, for this process to work, or even to have significant meaning, prerequisites for information must be met. Proper and adequate information must be effectively disseminated and made accessible to healthcare consumers, and channels of response or feedback, as well as their utilization must be made more effective. More will be said about this later.

An Overview of Some Healthcare Quality Measurement Issues

Healthcare quality monitoring efforts possess problems quite different from quality management in other sectors or industries of the economy, mainly because the routine assessment of healthcare quality has generally not been directly linked with the daily management of healthcare systems, the supply of healthcare services, and the day-to-day demand decisions for those services. It would be inconceivable to find that, for instance, electric appliance manufacturers and purchasers of their products did not immediately consider the quality of the product, and possibly that of related services (particularly when dealing with consumer durables) before or during conducting their transactions. Healthcare quality issues carry within themselves some fundamental questions which are not typical of quality issues in other sectors of the economy. Thus, the confidentiality and mutual trust upon which traditional patient-provider relationships have been based are not typical in most other buyer-seller relationships. On the other hand, the fear that some needed care may not be dispensed, or inexpensive care may be preferred over costly but superior care, because of healthcare cost containment efforts can find analogy in nonhealthcare sectors by way of cost-cutting efforts simply to increase profit margin.

To measure healthcare *quality*, it first has to be defined. That is, what are we trying to measure? The previous chapter dealt with these and related issues at some length. Suffice it here to simply review some of the basic premises, such as the notions of structure, process and outcome[2]. As we may recall, "structure" refers to the total composition of resources used to implement healthcare services, such as the staff, applied rules and regulations, and totality of physical facilities. "Process" is an intermediate output of care such as therapies, diagnostic and therapeutic procedures, utilization rate, and even access to particular care items. While "outcome" may be seen as the final products of care such as comfort, longevity including general health status, and patient satisfaction. As the complexity of medicine increases, so does the difficulty encountered when studying these three elements of health-care quality entity. In fact, for measurement purposes, structure and process may be helpful only if they can be meaningfully and causally linked to outcome. Otherwise, studies of the first two may be no more than exercises in futility and in the vacuum as far as healthcare quality measurements are concerned. That is perhaps the reason why attempts to measure healthcare quality have at times been related to efforts aimed at technology assessment, clinical evaluations, and randomized clinical trial - all structurally oriented areas of study.

Once defined, quality may be assessed or measured in various ways. The literature reflects on three broad categories: global direct, global indirect, and event-specific. *Global direct* approaches measurement problems by specifying direct criteria and then attempts somewhat mechanically to ascertain whether, based on available data and information, those criteria have been met. Standards are set and then evaluations are conducted to determine if and to what extent the standards are met. Criteria maps and criteria lists are established to determine if provider decisions at an early stage for recommending further care were in accordance with the set standards and criteria[3]. *Global indirect* measurements rely on external and presumably objective individual or group expert evaluations who assess in terms of their own judgment how well a provider, provider groups or provider systems have performed. Conclusions as to judgments and measurements of care quality implemented is usually arrived at by consensus[4]. Finally, *event-specific* measurements are based on predetermined procedures or practices that are considered undesirable or even harmful, and then contrast actual and carefully investigated specific care implementation events with these negative norms, encompassing various aspects of structure, process, and even outcome, within any single instance of care investigation[5]. There appear to be some inconsistencies in the results among the various methods. In particular, global direct and global indirect methods have yielded differing results in the same or similar situations, causing them to be favored by different interest groups within the medical profession: individual providers favoring the global indirect approach, while administrators and regulators favor the global direct method[6].

In the recent past much of the quality measurement efforts have concentrated on attempting to establish some causal relationships among the elements of quality, structure-process on the one hand and outcome on the other, often with the conclusion that structure and process individually or by bilaterally interact to generate some sort of outcome. In other words, a unilateral causal relationship was seen running from structure-process to outcome and care quality was finally seen as measurable in only terms of outcome, i.e. health status, comfort, functioning in society, and patient perception regarding the care. However, there are some potential problems particularly in the area of measurements, with this approach. We need to know some relevant production functions for care items to measure their outcome. If we know that function, then presumably any process may be used as a proxy for its predictable outcome, hence some sort of yardstick for that outcome, and vice versa. In the absence of a meaningful production function, however, an outcome, favorable or unfavorable, cannot be used as a measure or even an indicator of the quality of care service that goes into the process, hence useful managerial or policy decisions may be difficult or impossible to make. This discussion assumes, of course, that the pertinent production function in this context can utilize meaningfully some care service, care service component, or functionally meaningful care service groups as inputs for the generation of, again, some meaningful outcome (output), output component, or group of outcomes. In other words, both the input(s) and output(s), (the dependent and independent variables), are readily measurable for purposes of estimating and plotting the function. And, this is where much of the care quality measurement problem may rest.

Clearly, this analysis may also necessitate for us to know what elements of the healthcare service cause, if at all, what aspects of outcome. Does all or only some of implemented care generate the desired outcome or health status, all of that outcome, or part of it? What proportion, if any, of any given implemented healthcare process alters the interim and particularly the ultimate health status of the patient? And to what extent? The literature aimed even at the general non-medically trained public clearly indicates that with many medical problems, perhaps with a great majority of them in terms of their relative frequency of occurrence, some healthcare service implementations do little or nothing to alter the ultimate direction of the illness, i.e. its outcome for the patient. In most ambulatory circumstances, with uncompromised immune systems, illnesses tend to be self-limiting anyway, where care will have no impact on outcome and diagnostic or therapeutic medical efforts will likely add much more to healthcare costs than to the ultimate *physical* welfare of the patient. I emphasized "physical", because the visit to a provider might generate useful psychological assurances to effect of the absence of serious other medical problems [e.g. in the case of an otherwise normally self-curing common cold to rule out the presence of pneumonia]. If the patient's specific purpose is to simply rule out the much less likely major medical problems instead of seeking a "cure" for a common cold, then it may be argued that a visit to a primary care office is warranted and a production function might be constructed by way of using medical assurance as an input and some reassured state of patient mind as the output. But even without the obvious problems associated with measurability in this regard, to accommodate this type of analysis the concept of health outcome must be expanded well beyond its physical confines. Notions such as feelings, satisfaction, trust, attitude and a whole host of other abstract, intangible, and highly subjective factors need to be taken into consideration which may be almost impossible to define, let alone measure, even for one given patient let alone for a whole system of healthcare, and even for any given point in time let alone for various time periods involved.

We witness the marriage of art to science within medicine giving birth to virtually insurmountable problems in the way of meaningfully measuring healthcare quality, certainly by way of outcome. Thus, it may be that the separation of "outcome" from "process", in the objective Donebedian sense, in the eternal process of searching for healthcare quality measurements and risk assessment is highly unrealistic. It may also be that the results the patient is seeking, knowingly or unknowingly, in most cases are not even outcome, but rather the process itself, and the provider knows that that is exactly what he or she is producing, although the patient-provider interaction does not always reveal this predicament explicitly. It is, in turn, a process which generates its own *patient-specific outcome* of one kind or another, depending upon the specific patient's own input in terms of the earlier mentioned highly subjective and virtually nonmeasurable factors. Therefore, in this regard, the true and ultimate outcome will not be system-wide but patient-specific, causing further problems for system managers, healthcare policy researcher, healthcare evaluators, regulators and administrators.

The functional confusions in measuring quality reflect themselves in, and spills over into, the day-to-day administration of various quality related programs in hospital and other institutional provider settings. These programs are normally grouped into the following categories: "quality assurance" (QA), "risk management" (RM), and "utilization review" (UR), and their relationship to management's "total quality improvement" (TQI) programs. In particular, there appear to be questions as to the boundaries delineating the functions involved in QA, RM, and UR, and the manner whereby they may be arranged to reflect some hierarchical or time sequence relationships. For instance, a GAO report differentiates between RM and QA on the basis of their stated goals (RM - to prevent financial losses, and QA - to promote some optimum level of patient care). Yet, these functions often overlap obscuring the differences between their functions and even identity[7]. Thus, RM in minimizing negative financial outcome which is most likely to be caused by poor or negligent patient care, is often thought of as a QA territory. If we note that effective RM is also enhanced by effective problem preventive measures, then the demarcation between the two becomes even blurrier. This confusion might be mitigated somewhat by adding financial functions such as cost and insurance concerns to RM, but not to QA, and sequentially arranging their functions by viewing QA as a follow up to RM[8]. The so called Integrated Quality Assessment (IQA) is another approach which may functionally correlate QA, RM, and UR by integrating all care quality related functions, referring though mainly to the three traditional functions, i.e. QA, RM, and UR[9].

It appears that the confusion among the various quality related functions emanates from the fact that these functions are not distinct. Simply because institutional providers apply different working groups to these different functions does not mean that their functions are clearly differentiated. It is perhaps because of this predicament that the accrediting functions of the JCAHO are based largely on functions and specific processes aimed at quality improvement in a comprehensive and integrated context[10]. In addition to the various names, terms and definitions used by these different function groups for essentially the same thing, separated focus on quality and cost control is not clear, duplicative and often redundant data collection and data utilization takes place, and there is a frequent lack of coordination among these and related activities. Furthermore, these functions even within a hospital are narrowly focused, applied to small specific areas of various endeavors which may not communicate with each other[11]. The introduction of some other control functions such as total quality improvement (TQI) and total quality management (TQM) does not seem to clear up the confusion; perhaps on the contrary. These additional functions are essentially data-based management change and improvement tools, relying most upon data and information banks collected from past customers of the provider, and thus attempting to improve care quality[12]. Furthermore, in some circles TQI is seen as a replacement for QA and UR since the former is seen as a replacement rendering the latter two functions as redundant[13].

Regulation, Quasi-Regulation and Databases

These dimensions are spread over office-based, hospital-based, and home care environments both for institutional and private providers. The broadest form of quality enforcement is probably implemented through accrediting and licensing providers. *Accreditation* of hospitals is done mostly voluntarily by the Joint Commission for the Accreditation of Healthcare Organizations (JCAHO). Of the 7000 or so hospitals that participate in Medicare, over three-quarters sought and received JCAHO accreditation. These constitute hospitals with over 50 beds, leaving mostly rural smaller hospitals in the unaccredited areas. The method of accreditation incorporates elaborate self-assessment procedures as well as tri-annual on-site surveys of three days duration utilizing a specific scoring procedure. Full or contingent accreditation is given, with the latter convertible into the former, upon completion of certain requirements[14]. Until 1981, the JCAHO appeared to require the maintenance of specific structure-based standards, however, it was subsequently replaced to some extent by a perpetual process of care monitoring, while retaining structural consideration only to ensure a care environment consistent with prescribed quality, such as the requirement that a quality assurance program be implemented by medical staff, and that provisions be made for the continuous evaluation of the medical staff[15].

The JCAHO's accreditation efforts may yield important care quality indicators if the standards are uniformly and consistently applied. In fact, JCAHO generated quality indicators could be important factors to consider when comparing various hospitals. JCAHO accreditation could also be considered by third-party payers and outside regulators. This is notwithstanding the fact that accreditation is voluntarily sought by hospitals, and that the evaluation process may be viewed as an internal one to the hospitals for the JCAHO itself is constituted by its hospital members to whom, therefore, it is presumably accountable. In general, accreditation means that certain quality assurance efforts such as desirable staffing policies, credential monitoring, and proper internal grievance procedures are in place. In other words, at least the care structure for a quality oriented care process is implemented, but with no necessary further monitoring of the outcome. Finally, and without meaning to imply a criticism of that process, there does not appear to be in place any mechanism whereby the evaluation process itself is monitored with respect to its own quality and reliability. We might also add here that in addition to the JCAHO, there are other accrediting agencies such as the Accreditation Association for Ambulatory Health Care (AAAHC), the

National Committee on Quality Assurance (NCQA) for HMO's, and the National League for Nursing (NLN) for home health agencies. They too function upon the invitation of the organization that seeks to be accredited, and while their activities seem to be increasing in some states such as Pennsylvania and Kansas, they have been relatively passive in the past.

In addition to accreditation, credentialing by way of *certification* by subspeciality and speciality boards, and licensing by state boards can play an important role in quality enforcement. Physicians are certified by some 23 speciality boards recognized by the American Board of Medical Specialities (ABMS). Thus, "board certification" means that by the ABMS, more than other smaller entities that also certify physicians, although many physicians designate themselves as specialist without having any certification. Members from AMA and the ABMS make up the Accreditation Council for Graduate Medical Education (ACGME) which approves residency programs. As an index of care quality, certification has been recognized as significant, and certification verification can be obtained from the AMA (Physician Master File, and American Medical Directory), and the ABMS[16]. Whether or not there are significant differences between board certified and non-certified specialists in terms of some quality care criteria is questionable. Professional ratings, medical record-based performance evaluations, and patient satisfaction yardsticks suggest no significant care quality differences between the two groups. It has been found that board certification, while may suggest in some cases superior process, assures no superior quality of care in terms of outcome in comparison with care rendered by non-certified specialist. Furthermore, such care quality related conclusions can only be drawn in one speciality at a time, and any care quality conclusion with respect to one area of specialization may not readily be applied to other areas[17].

States are responsible for *licensing* their medical providers, legally precluding those who are not licensed from practice. State boards of medical examiners issue licenses based on education, experience, training, personal attributes, and a variety of other factors. Licenses are reciprocally recognized by some of the states. However, while licensing does meet some minimum quality standards, it does not satisfy most quality assurance provisions. In addition, once the license is granted, it is good for life and is not significantly threatened even when periodic competence tests are applied. Its utilization by the practitioner is substantively constrained only by criminal statutes and civil malpractice contingencies[18].

Beyond these largely statutorily based measures of attempt to assure some minimum standard for care quality, there are some less formal ones applied in various forms at different types of institution. Thus, so called practice guidelines (sometimes also labeled as "patient care algorithms") may be used to ensure some minimum quality standards, or for standards against which the quality of performed services may be tested. These guidelines are a systemic, often graphic and charted, presentation of medical textbook principles based on scientific evidence as well as on clinical experience. If they are updated for changes in the state of the art, and also made adaptable for complex and multiple patient conditions, they have been thought of as useful tools for securing some standards of healthcare quality. A junior cousin of practice guidelines is the "clinical reminder system" (frequently used in managed care environments, clinics and private office practices) which indicates preventive tests, drug interactions and laboratory tests for some specific cases encountered by the provider. If provided through elaborate and efficient computer and related database systems, and if the provider has the computer facilities and resources (particularly time) to utilize them in a timely fashion during office-hours while the patient is present, this process can be helpful in maintaining minimum quality standards[19].

There are various databases available for possible care quality assessments. These include datasets on Medicare A and B claims, hospitals discharge abstracts, patient identifying numbers, and health program enrollment particulars. Data of this sort can be used for geographical and time-based inpatient mortality studies, lengths of stays, hospital specific readmission instances, long-term outcome surveys, and variety of other patient specific and population-based studies. In addition, ambulatory care datasets can shed light on the rate of hospitalization, readmissions, and the stage at which a disease is first diagnosed[20]. These and other similar data sources are almost readily available to those who wish to perform studies, for clinical decision making, risk assessment procedures, tracking outcomes and so forth. Their utility, however, is limited by the extent to which the data are correct and complete, and the degree to which the procedure coding system utilized in the datasets is explicit enough to reveal needed data in an unbundled form.

Broad Negative Quality Indices

There is a large number of accountable opportunities in medicine for quality problems to occur in the structure, process or outcome areas, if clearly demarcated, and in other less demarcated areas of medical endeavor which may not clearly fall into these three traditional areas of quality components.

Thus, by way of a scenario, it does not happen very infrequently where a patient with a normally terminal cancer or another type of normally terminal disease is told that he/she has 3-6 months to live, only to find that the patient will have survived for 5 years or more. What medical care quality connotations would one want to attach to those situations? A superficial response would be, "great" it is a pleasant surprise and make the most of it. Thus, outcome clearly does not indicate a negative quality although the professional prediction of outcome was inaccurate. On the other hand, if the patient acted on that prediction, for instance by way of a suicide, or extreme depression, or by making unwarranted arrangements in his or her own personal or financial affairs in anticipation of death, then the positive outcome (which may not even be an outcome pursuant any specific medical structure or process) is at best tempered, and may even be completely offset, by a negative reaction to a harmful medical prediction. It is possible that this type of care, and malfeasance in it (given that the providers themselves may genuinely be surprised by the outcome based on historical statistics pertaining to the disease, its labeling as a "malfeasance" may also be tenuous) would fall into what has traditionally been called technical and interpersonal care category. This category then is clearly a likely one where negative quality dimensions may be identified. There may be at least two others, not necessarily clearly demarcated or demarcable from technical competence, entailing the extent to which by way of process the existing structures are utilized: *excessive and deficient utilization*. Thus, the latter two while quality embedded, clearly have cost implications as well.

The *technical qualities* of care considerations are normally included in procedures such as diagnosis, prescribed medication, and surgical procedures where applicable. Since the process intensively involves dealing and interacting with the patient personally, it includes a subcategory of technical qualities by way of *interpersonal skills* (effectively communicating with the patient prior to process items to enable the patient to make informed decisions about treatment alternatives, if possible during, and subsequent to any of these process items to enable the patient to follow treatment plans). While interpersonal care aspects of the process are clearly important, it appears as we noted earlier that quality assurance programs tend to concentrate on technical quality related variables instead of interpersonal issues, such as skill implementation, performance indicators, operational system functioning, surgical review, morbidity, and other adverse events.

Technical quality assessments may point to practitioners with negative notoriety or to problems with entire care systems within hospitals. Yet, private or institutional providers with negative notoriety in a given area need not be assumed to lack technical qualities in all areas, as the finding of negative performance indicators at one time does not necessarily suggest permanent problems. For instance, hospital-specific mortality data generated by the HCFA (discussed earlier in the volume) rarely points to institutional providers with high mortalities in all or most areas of their endeavors, and to institutions whose high mortality rates persist over a number of years. On the other hand, it may also be validly argued (and medical malpractice data have suggested) that providers with a generally positive performance track record need not be assumed to be flawless in all aspects of their processes at all times.

The technical quality of care is normally assessed based on research literature, disciplinary actions, or medical malpractice data. One such *research study* used Medical Management Analysis data which reported adverse patient occurrences [unexpected and abnormal consequence of the patient's disease or applied procedure] with about one out of every five admitted hospital patients. The same study also looked at peer-approved surgeons, based on patient charts, and revealed that in one out of four cases there was at least one such adverse patient occurrence. On an individual surgeon basis, adverse patient occurrences ranged from about 20% to about 30% and seemed to vary directly with the complexity of cases involved[21]. Another study reported on a review by three or more physicians of 183 death cases and found that almost 10% of the deaths could have been preventable, hence were due to errors in management or diagnosis, although the reasons varied by type of admission[22]. Yet a third study compared practice performance as indicated by charts with those standards which the compared practitioners themselves have set and found considerable deviations of actual practice from the peer-set standards. Thus, using antibiotic applications in a community hospital, on the average, only about 50% of the antibiotic applications were up to or above the standards set within the hospital itself[23].

State medical board reports pursuant to *disciplinary actions* can reflect on medical competence. The frequency of these actions tend to vary by state ranging from 0 to 15 per 1,000 practitioners, with a national average rate of about 4.5 per 1,000 practitioners. According to the Federation of State Licensing Boards (FSLB), some 2,300 disciplinary actions were taken nationally against a half-million practitioners in 1986. The outcome of these actions may range from license revocation, suspension, probation down through letters of reprimands and informal communications[24]. Physician owned insurance companies were forced to terminate coverage for about 7 practitioners per thousand due to negligent behavior, and to restrict coverage for about that many again because of less than adequate care when compared to accepted standards[25]. Malfeasances related to technical competence tended to center on faulty prescription writing, particularly for those involving controlled substances, and substance (drug, alcohol) abuse by the practitioner himself/herself. Non-technical competence related violations heard by state disciplinary boards included insurance fraud, professional misconduct and felony violations[26].

As to using medical *malpractice data* as a yardstick for technical competence, the picture is blurry at best. Earlier in the volume, I have discussed at some length the problems involved with the reliability of malpractice judgments and settlement amounts for measuring the severity of malfeasance, or problems with technical performance, if any. But apart from the reliability problems associated with the outcome of those claims, many malfeasances are simply not claimed for. A comparison of the so called "potentially compensable events" (PCEs) in the California Medical Insurance Feasibility (CMIF) database with actual insurance claims suggests that no more than 10% of potentially valid claims are actually brought to any form of litigation. Based on a 100% increase in claims since the CMIF data was compiled, a more recent study suggested a corresponding 20% factor. The same study found that about 1% of hospital admissions yielded negative events of various degrees for the patients involved[27]. Thus, apart from the severe reliability problems associated with using the outcomes (whatever that may be) of medical malpractice litigation as a measure of the nature or degree of malfeasance on the part of medical defendants, an overwhelming majority of malfeasances instances are not even litigated or claimed for in any form in the first place. Reiterating in sum and substance of what we already stated with respect to medical malpractice litigation outcomes, whether in the form of jury verdict, judge's judgment, or settlements at various stages of the litigation, the amount with which the litigation is concluded cannot even remotely be thought of as an indicator of the magnitude of the malpractice and therefore the negative quality of the care involved in the incident. A judgment, verdict, or settlement in a medical malpractice litigation is some culmination of the interaction of personalities, legal skills or lack thereof, political, economic and social value judgments, biases, professional diligence or lack thereof, psychological states of mind, and a whole host of other non-measurable and noncontrollable factors which may render the verdict, judgment, or settlement unrecognizable and indeed meaningless in relation to the assessment of a possible medical malfeasance that might have been involved. Notwithstanding this posture on the part of the author, it behooves us to reflect on some of the more formal studies that have been done in this regard[28].

In addition to problems indicated above, malpractice claims, perhaps because of the small proportion of possible provider malfeasances that are formally complained or claimed against, have tended to target a relatively small proportion of provider population. Thus, studies have shown that in Michigan, for instance, less than 3% of the practicing physicians were targeted by almost one-fifth of the claims, in other words every fifth claim was aimed at that small proportion of practitioners. The concentration is further magnified by noting that some 20% of physicians were responsible for over 70% of all claims. In Florida, during the decade following 1974, over half of "medmal" claims were paid on behalf of some 50% of the practicing physicians (probably mostly OB/GYN specialists)[29]. Apart from the earlier indicated problems with medical malpractice claims paid, even less reliance can be placed on just claims alone without at least some indications as to how the claims were resolved. A national study found that in 1984 over half of the claims were dismissed without any financial remedy for the claimant[30]. Apparently over two-thirds of the claims were targeted against physicians, some 20% against hospitals, with the rest against other healthcare professionals and allied healthcare employees. Finally, it should be pointed out with regards to malpractice claims as a possible yardstick for care quality measurements that it would be just as faulty to conclude that there are necessarily no care quality problems with those providers who were *not* targeted with malpractice claim(s) as to conclude that all of those against whom claims were targeted are necessarily inferior performers not only in the long-run but even with respect to the claimed instance.

Informed judgments regarding certain aspects of care quality may also be formed based on *excessive utilization* of available facilities. "Excessive" in this context may be defined as an increment in service utilization which yields a negative net utility for the patient. In other words, the additional service does more harm than good, that is, the likelihood of morbidity or mortality exceeds that of an improvement in health status. This may apply to diagnostic services where frequently occurring false "positives" or "high" readings (e.g. PSA tests for prostate cancer) can lead to a chain of likely unnecessary but consequent tests and procedures (e.g. transrectal ultrasound examinations and biopsies of the prostate), or antibiotic prescriptions where excessive utilization may render the patient vulnerable to antibiotic resistant bacteria. Finally, the direct economic consequences of excessive utilization may be noted in terms of the opportunity cost incurred by society if the extra amount of resources taken up by excessive utilization are diverted from other more vital opportunities, and in terms of explicit costs measured simply in terms of the moneys spent on the unnecessary utilization.

Yet, excessive utilization is difficult to avoid in our society. In general, the motto "when in doubt, you act" is imbedded in our thinking. We want to be certain that "there is really nothing wrong", often in spite of asymptomatic conditions. Physician's fear, or at least apprehension, of malpractice claims also often mandates prudence by acting rather than not acting when it comes to testing and diagnostics ("defensive medicine"). However, even under those circumstances, it would be very difficult to draw a line between necessary and prudent care, and over utilization of the type being discussed here. If anything goes wrong, the "should haves" or "could haves" will likely dominate. A response during a malpractice trial "I did not think at that time that it was necessary" with reference to a test or diagnostic procedure will not carry much weight in favor of the physician. Thus, the dilemma is serious. While it is easy to theorize and analyze issues about excessive utilization in a scholarly context, it is a difficult matter to look at in the actual practice and circumstances of the physician. When one looks further at these issues in our technologically enhanced environment where the most modern tools of accurate and non-invasive diagnostics are at the ready disposal of the physician and the patient, "excessive utilization" becomes even more difficult to delineate. Nevertheless, studies have been done to measure the extent of excessive utilization, some of which have found evidence of it in areas of diagnostic tests, hospital inpatient care, and various surgical procedures. Almost 20% of upper GI, and the same proportion of coronary angiography, and some 15% of coronary bypass procedures were found to be unnecessary. Similar excessive utilization was found with EKGs, colonoscopies and sigmoidoscopies, prostatectomies, and some other procedures[31].

On the opposite side of the picture, "*deficient utilization*" may also be seen by some as a care quality indicator. It can be defined as the difference between proper utilization and some lesser amount that has in fact been implemented, where this difference would have yielded a net benefit for the patient, independent of the marginal explicit and opportunity costs that would have been incurred had this additional service been performed. Since this is a forgone event or events, i.e. something that has not taken place, its measurement tends to be somewhat more convoluted than that of excessive utilization. These deficiencies may occur due either to a lack of access to care or to a nonperformance of diagnostic or therapeutic care service items by providers. The latter have often been alleged in medical malpractice suits.

Thus, when access to care is not an issue, these deficiencies may occur due to sheer negligence, mistaken diagnoses, or possibly by design brought about by financial incentives in managed care environments. The latter will be dealt with more extensively later in this volume.

In more clinical contexts, some physicians have developed a set of institutionally based negative quality signs which enumerated in relatively recent literature. The following are some of those negative indicators: (a) Patients are discharged directly from hospital intensive care units (ICUs) to their homes, instead of to gradually lower levels of care within the hospital or affiliated institutions has been seen as a negative indicator of quality. In this regards good relationship with skilled nursing care facilities should be sought after. (b) Excess usage of ICU facilities may be found under circumstances where criteria for admitting and transferring patients have not been set. (c) Overutilized telemetry beds can result in reduced cost effectiveness and misallocation of facilities among patients needing monitored beds. (d) Errors and mix-ups are more likely in formularies which carry all FDA approved drugs in contrast to those which carry only those most important for the hospital. (e) Unnecessary and extra days of post surgical antibiotics exposure may result from a lack of automatic stop orders with the prescriptions involved. (f) Without adequate discharge planning, patients may stay in the hospital environment longer than necessary exposing them additional adverse events. (g) Medical staff should be represented on the PRO so as to communicate findings directly back to the hospital environment. (h) Quality control by the credentialing process may be indicated by the frequency with which medical staff applications are rejected at the hospital. (i) Various procedures need to be in place to ensure that physicians sign their charts, hence proper accountability may be assigned. (j) The quality of medical chart and record composition may be an indication of the attention that the physician pays to the case[32]. However, although all these may be warning signs, they are imbedded in care structure and process with little or nothing to offer directly in outcome. The author is not aware of any studies which meaningfully linked these and other similar quality warning signs with care outcomes.

Notes

1.   A later chapter in this volume will be devoted entirely to this issue.
2.   See references to Donabedian, A., "Evaluating the Quality of Care", *Milbank Memorial Fund Quarterly,* Vol. 44, July 1966 (Part II); by the same author, *Explorations in Quality Assessment and Monitoring,* Vol. I: The Definition of Quality and

Approaches to its Assessment, Health Administration Press, Ann Arbor, MI 1980; and, Vol. I *The Criteria and Standards of Quality*, same publisher, 1982; also by the same author, *The Methods and Findings of Quality Assessment and Monitoring: An Illustrated Analysis*, same publisher, 1985.

3. Payne, B., Lyons, T., Dwarshius, L. et al., *The Quality of Medical Care: Evaluation and Improvement*, Hospital Research and Educational Trust, Chicago, IL, 1976. See also, Greenfield, S., Lewis, C.E., Kaplan, S.H. et al., "Peer Review by Criteria Mapping: Criteria for Diabetes Mellitus: The Use of Decision Making in Chart Audit", Annals of Internal Medicine, Vol. 83, 1975; and, Greenfield, S., Cretin, S. and Wortham, L. et al., "Comparison of a Criteria Map to a Criteria List in Quality of Care Assessment for Patients with Chest Pain: The Relation of Each to Outcome", *Medical Care*, Vol. 19, March 1981. Some of the relevant basic issues are discussed in Lembcke, P.A., "Evolution of Medical Audit", *JAMA*, Vol. 199, February 1967; Brook, R.H., "Critical Issues in the Assessment of Quality-of-Care and Their Relationship to HMOs", *Journal of Medical Education*, Vol. 48, 1973; Brook, R.H. and Appel, F.A., "Quality of Care Assessment: Choosing a Method for Peer Review", *New England Journal of Medicine*, Vol. 288, 1973.

4. Moorehead, M.A., Donaldson, R.S. et al., "A Study of the Quality of Hospital Care Secured by a Sample of Teamster Family Members in New York City", Columbia University, School of Public Health, New York, 1964; and Moorehead, M.A., "The Medical Audit as an Operational Tool", *American Journal of Public Health*, Vol. 57, 1967. See also Hulka, B.S., Romm, F.J., Parkerson, G.R. et al., "Peer Review in Ambulatory Care: Use of Explicit Criteria and Implicit Judgement", *Medical Care*, Vol. 17 (Supp), Vol. 1, 1979.

5. Rutstein, D.D., Berenberg, W., Chalmers, T.C. et al., "Measuring the Quality of Medical Care: A Clinical Method", *New England Journal of Medicine*, Vol. 294, 1976. Ciocco, A. et al., "Statistics on the Clinical Services to New Patients in Medical Groups", *Public Health Reports*, Vol. 65, 1950; and Ciocco, A., "On Indeces for the Appraisal of Health Department Activities", *Journal of Chronic Diseases*, Vol. 11, 1960; Sheps, M.C., "Approached to the Quality of Hospital Care", *Public Health Reports*, Vol. 70, 1955.

6. See Hulka, Romm et al. cited above.

7. General Accounting Office, *Healthcare Initiatives in Hospital Risk Management*, Washington, DC, 1989, HRD-89-79.

8. Molnagle, J.F., *Risk Management: A Guide for Healthcare Professionals*, Aspen Publishing, Rockville, MD, 1985. See also Bloom, A., *The Role of Risk Management in the Assessment of the Quality of Care in HMOs*, Proceeding of the 37th Annual Group Health Institute. Group Health Association of America, Seattle, WA, 1987.

9. Longo, D.R., Ciccone, K.R., Lord, J.T., *Integrated Quality Assessment: A Model for Concurrent Review*, American Hospital Publishing, Chicago, IL, 1989.

10. Joint Commission On Accreditation of Healthcare Organizations, *Joint Commission Agenda for Change: Indicator Development and Testing*, Chicago, IL, 1991.

11. See Longo et al.

12. Smith, D.G., Wheeler, J.R.C., "Strategies and Structures for Hospital Risk Management Programs", *Healthcare Management Review*, Vol. 17, 1992.

13. See JCAHO note#10.

14. The discussion of the detailed and specific medically technical requirements to be met by the candidate institution is beyond the scope of this volume.

15. JCAHO, *Accreditation Manual for Hospitals* (AMH), Vol. I & II, Chicago, IL, 1994. See also JCAHO, *Making Accreditation Decisions for Hospitals*, 1994; JCAHO *Score 100: A Tool for Predicting Survey Outcomes*, 1994; in addition, for general

information, refer to JCAHO's internally generated informational bulletins: *Facts About the Joint Commission* - 1994, *Joint Commission History* - 1994, *Joint Commission's Confidentiality and Discloure Policy* - 1994, *The Agenda for Change* - 1994, *The Joint Commission's Performance Measurement Initiative* - 1994, *Background on Health Care Quality* - 1994, *Joint Commission Survey and Accreditation Process* - 1994, and *Questions & Answers, Performance Measures* - 1994.

16. JCAHO Publications. Also see Davis, D., Haynes, R.B. et al., "The Impact of CME: A Methodologic Review of the Continuing Medical Education Literature", *Evaluation and the Health Professions*, Vol. 7, 1984. Havinghurst, C.C., *Healthcare Law and Policy: Readings, Notes and Questions*, Foundation Press, Westbury, NY, 1988; and Havinghurst, C.C., King, N.M., "Private Credentialing of Healthcare Personnel: An Antitrust Perspective", *American Journal of Law & Medicine*, Vol. 9, 1983.

17. Office of Technology Assessment, *The Quality of Care, Information for Consumers*, OTA-H-386 GPO, Washington, DC, 1988. Ramsey, P.G. et al., "Predictive Validity of Certification by the American Board of Internal Medicine, *Annals of Internal Medicine*, Vol. 110, 1989.

18. See Davis and also Havinghurst.

19. Tierney, W.M. et al., "Delayed Feedback of Physician Performance Versus Immediate Reminders to Perform Preventive Care: Effects on Physician Compliance", *Medical Care*, Vol. 24, 1986. See also Barnett, G.O. et al., "Quality Assurance Through Automated Monitoring and Concurrent Feedback Using a Computer-Based Medical Information System", *Medical Care*, Vol. 16, 1978.

20. Weiner, J. et al., *Quality of Care Indicators for Potential Application to Insurance Claims/Encounter Data*, Report to the Cigna Foundation. John Hopkins University Research and Development Center, Baltimore, MD, 1989. See also, Roos, L.L. et al., "Risk Adjustment in Claim-based Research: The Search for Efficient Approaches", *Journal of Clinical Epidemiology*, Vol. 42, 1989.

21. Cradic, J.W. and Bader, B.S., *Medical Management Analysis, A Systemic Approach to Quality Assurance and Risk Management*, Vol. I, Auburn, CA, 1983.

22. Dubois, R.W. and Brook, R.H., "Preventable Deaths: Who, How Often, and Why?", *Annals of Internal Medicine*, Vol. 109, 1988.

23. Jogerts, G.L. and Dippe, S.E., "Antibiotic Use Among Medical Specialists", *JAMA*, Vol. 245, 1981.

24. Office of Technology Assessment, *The Quality of Medical Care. Information for Consumers*, OTA-H-386, USGPO, Washington, DC, 1988.

25. Wolfe, S.M. (ed), "State Medical Board Doctor Disciplinary Actions: 1987", *The Public Citizen Health Research Group Health Letter*, Vol. 5, 1989.

26. Office of Inspector General, Department of Health and Human Services, *Medical Licensure and Discipline: An Overview*, Department of Health and Human Services P-ol-86-0064, Office of Analysis and Inspection, Washington, DC, 1986. See also Derbyshire, R.C., *Medical Discipline in Disarray: Retrospective and Prospective Hospital Practice*, Vol. 19, 1984. Derbyshire claimed at that time that some 10% of individual medical practitioners were professionally incompetent to practice, where professional incompetence was defined as a physician's inability to satisfactorily care for patients due to faulty judgements professional absolescence, unavailability, and general unreliability for whatever reasons within the practitioner's control.

27. Mills, D.H. (ed), *Report on the Medical Insurance Feasibility Study*, California Medical Association and California Hospital Association, San Francisco, CA, 1977. Danzon, P.M., *Medical Malpractice: Theory, Evidence and Public Policy*, Harvard University Press, Cambridge, MA, 1985.

28. The author has functioned as an economic expert witness in a substantial number of medical malpractice cases with various types of plaintiffs and defendants, their lawyers of considerable heterogeneity, insurers, other third parties, in various parts of the US, during the past twenty years, and has gained an intimate and an extensive amount of hopefully reliable knowledge of the roles, motives, skills, performances, techniques, and a whole host of other dimensions and aspects regarding the actors and the outcomes that are involved in these largely economically motivated dramas. See also Office of Technology Assessment. *The Quality of Medical Care. Information for Consumers.* OTA-H-386, GPO, Washington, DC, 1988.

29. Wolfe, S.M., Testimony Before Civil and Constitutional Rights Subcommittee, House Judiciary Committee, October, 1986.

30. General Accounting Office, *Medical Malpractice: Characteristics of Claims Closed in 1984*, HDR-87-55, GPO, Washington, DC, 1987.

31. Brown, R.E., Sheingold, S.H. and Luce, B.R., *Options of Using Practice Guidelines in Reducing the Volume of Medically Unnecessary Services* BHARC-013/89/027, Battelle Human Affairs Research Centers, Washington, DC, 1989; Park, R.E., Fink, A. et al., *Physician Ratings of Appropriate Indications for Six Medical and Surgical Procedures,* R-3280-CWF/HF/PMT/RWJ, The Rand Corporation, Santa Monica, CA, 1986; Brook, R.H., Lohr, K.N., "Will We Need to Ration Effective Healthcare?", *Issues in Science and Technology,* Vol. 3, Fall 1986; Winslow, C.M., Kosecoff, J.B., Chassin, M.R. et al., "The Appropriateness of Performing Coronary By-Pass Surgery", *JAMA,* Vol. 260, 1988, and using essentially the same methodology, Winslow, C.M., Solomon, D.H., Chassin, M.R. et al., "The Appropriateness of Carotid Endarterectomy", *New England Journal of Medicine,* Vol. 318, 1988; Merrick, N.K., Brook, R.H., Fink, A. et al., "Use of Carotid Endarterectomy in Five California Veterans Administration Hospitals", *JAMA,* Vol. 258, 1986.

32. Musfeldt, C., "Twenty-Five Warning Signs of Quality Problems", *Hopitals,* January 5, 1991.

5 Measuring Healthcare Quality: Empiricisms

We have remarked earlier that indications of healthcare quality problems, indeed the reasons for hospital inpatient morbidity and mortality are the occurrence and recurrence of so-called adverse events, much of it by way of internally acquired infections. In order to assess the empirical weight that may be given to this type of negative occurrence in hospital environments, a study was conducted recently in New York State. The researchers estimated that about 4% of hospitalized patients in New York experienced some type of significant negative occurrence in 1984[1]. These negative occurrences were viewed as those caused in some way by a provider resulting in measurable disability. The study involved some 30,000 randomly selected hospital records in New York State during 1984, of which about 1,100 showed some type of negative occurrence. Of these negative occurrences, some 28% were found to be due to negligence and 42% due to non-negligence based errors. Over 66% of these were viewed as preventable errors. The errors included technical ones while performing operations, procedures or tests (44%), those in diagnosis (17%), failure to prevent negative occurrences (12%), and drug prescription problems (10%). Most of the preventable errors (60%) occurred in the broad categories of general medicine and general surgery. In terms of preventability, there was no significant difference found between hospital and ambulatory settings, however, within hospitals emergency room-based errors were found to be more preventable than those occurring elsewhere, while in environments external to hospitals free-standing ambulatory surgical units seemed most vulnerable to preventable errors.

The study further found that 78% of the fatal *errors* were preventable, although it may not follow that the same proportion of the *deaths* caused by preventable errors were themselves also preventable. In other words, it was not ascertained that in case of each mortality, a non-occurrence of the preventable error would have also enabled the patient to survive the illness involved, i.e. the death itself would have been preventable. The errors in general are attributed to the complexities of modern highly technical invasive medicine such as those applied in cardiac, vascular and neuro surgeries, and to the high volume of care items in some respects, such as in medications[2].

The Uniform Clinical Data Set System (UCDSS) and Other Health Databases

The recently evolved drive to contain medical costs gave rise to concerns for care quality. The later, in turn, caused the implementation of various care monitoring processes by governments, hospital administrations, third-party payers, and various managed care organizations. As part of the government's concern for this trade-off between care costs and care quality, the Health Care Financing Administration developed the UCDSS as a computerized system of methods designed to monitor healthcare quality, mainly for peer review organizations (PROs). It was first tested in 1991 in five states, and is expected to be fully implemented by mid-1995. At this point, we will examine this system in terms of its more general dimensions. In Chapter 8, some of the specific HFCA databases and files will be reviewed.

The UCDSS is essentially a computer program which allows the performance of three basic functions: abstraction of medical records by way of data entry from patient charts, the application of a set of rules (algorithms) to evaluate the care indicated on each chart, an assessment of the total care process subsequent to discharge[3]. The abstraction phase normally entails basic data regarding the case such as patient biographical and physician identifications, admission source, medical history and physical examination, prevailing functional status, diagnostic findings by way of laboratory, imaging, and endoscopic tests and procedures, treatment interventions such as medications, possible medical complications, and discharge status. The algorithms in turn, applied to the case abstracts, attempt to ascertain the need for hospital admissions, the quality of inpatient care, and discharge management related issues. The final output of the UCDSS is a clinical abstract which, while less detailed than the patient's chart, enables care quality evaluators to efficiently assess the care process.

While the system was developed for external reviews conducted by PROs, it has been found to have some actual uses for hospital inpatient care assessments. However, with the latter option some problems were discovered relating mainly to the time and effort costs involved with the initial abstraction process, and to the frequency of errors in assessments which this relatively automatic system may generate[4]. Perhaps because of these problems, and due to a change in orientation from specific case reviews to more general data collection and analyses systems to support PROs, the UCDSS is being transformed into a so-called Medicare Quality Indicator System (MQIS). These concentrate more on profiling care processes and outcomes than analyzing specific cases. In particular, the MQIS methodology will develop disease-specific quality indicators in order to profile patterns of care for providers. These quality indicators will follow published guidelines or accepted standards of care and will be backed by appropriate and continuously collected data. This change by HCFA from the originally devised UCDSS system to MQIS was apparently brought about by changes in the application and utilization of PRO programs under the Healthcare Quality Improvement Act. The change appears to scrap much of previously collected actual data under UCDSS, although experiences and problems recognized under the previous data collection (abstraction) processes, particularly in terms of efficiency and accuracy related problems, will apply under the new system[5].

In addition to the UCDSS/MQIS, other datasets and databases are emerging which are designed to monitor and improve the delivery of healthcare quality. The development of mass storage and fast retrieval yet compact and efficient datahandling systems, the opportunity is emerging to gather, process, and disseminate healthcare quality related information regarding individual as well as institutional providers. Broad population-based databases on all of those who procured any healthcare services, and the many possible dimensions (fields) for the records in those databases, allow for an unprecedented banking of relevant information regarding healthcare services throughout the profession and populations. However, as with many other databased and personally related information, a trade-off emerges: the dangers of invading the privacy of patients and providers vs. the benefits of such invasion for members of society as a whole. Yet, an Institute of Medicine Committee, using the term regional *health database organization* (HDO) envisions these databases as containing patient-specific data outside the immediate care environment, also reporting about providers, and released to the public[6]. We will note later in the volume, however, that some of the HCFA databases and files are in fact inaccessible to the public.

Empirical Issues in Outcome Assessment

Assessing quality in terms of outcomes may be viewed as assessing outcomes in relation to some standard(s), and, therefore, in some respects to assess variations within outcome groups or occurrences. A derivative question relates to how much variation, or how much of the variations, in outcomes may be attributed to particular individual or institutional practice styles, instead of to other factors. Treatment outcome (TO) may be a function of a number of factors, such as patient personality and ability (or willingness) to communicate symptoms (P), initial patient condition (C_i) diagnostic (D), treatment (T) and follow-up treatment (T_f) procedures undertaken by providers, patient-specific reaction (R) to the treatment, where the latter depends on that patient's bio-medical characteristics and the nature as well as timing of the treatment[7], TO = $f(P,C_i,D,T,R,T_f)$. Increasing system capacities to measure and compute will make this type of complex approaches possible.

Yet, I must note that the complexity increases with the recognition that outcomes themselves need interpretation in terms of their status within the treatment process. Some outcomes can be considered intermediate and only some others as final, meaning different things to patients and providers. In connection with the treatment of heart ailments, *biochemical* outcomes (decreased serum lactate or natriuretic hormonc levels), *physiological* outcomes (decreased systemic vascular resistance), *anatomical* outcomes (decreased heart size or reduced coronary artery obstruction) and *histological* outcomes (reduced myocardial hypertrophy) may all be considered as intermediate outcomes of major significance to the physician, but of little immediate or ultimate concern to the patient. *Clinical* outcome (reduced mortality, improved physical functioning, reduced symptoms), on the other hand, may be considered as final outcome of significance to the patient as well as to the physician. Clearly, mortality or lack thereof is the ultimate outcome in terms of some objective evaluation, although may not be the most desirable as a yardstick for monitoring the effectiveness of a treatment ("too much or too little recognized too late"). An assessment of the patient's initial risk of death and how specific treatment alternatives affect that risk are of more immediate concern for the provider at the time of coming into contact with the patient. When the clinical outcome of mortality occurs, it is obviously too late. On the other hand, from the physician's point of view mortality risks can also be assessed from intermediate outcomes, and risks or predictions of mortality at those stages of the treatment process can scientifically be ascertained[8].

Whatever levels of outcome may be considered as inputs for care quality measurements, some sort of *risk-adjustment* needs to be applied. This becomes particularly important when outcomes data, such as mortality, are published for potential consumers of care. Business and insurance groups would tend to avoid high negative outcome providers, on the one hand, and providers to protect their reputation would tend to avoid caring for patients who are perhaps in the greatest need for urgent care, the high risk ones. Thus, effective risk-adjustments control for severity differences among patients, and attempt to generate standards upon which care quality can be meaningfully compared without risk biases, and care costs can by themselves be considered when choosing a provider of equal or different quality level. The implementation of effective risk adjustment system requires data, such as computer processed discharge information, abstracted from original medical records. The process is cumbersome, difficult and was relatively slow getting underway. The first state mandating systematic data collection was Pennsylvania in 1986, prompted largely by business concerns for severity measurements. It involves massive clinical abstraction efforts from medical records, which upon processing, is designed for public release[9]. However, in spite of various and spreading state efforts to generate data which may facilitate risk-adjustments and possibly care quality evaluations, it still seems confusing whether or not risk adjusted data can be used for quality comparisons, and it may not even be always clear what the risk-adjusted data actually means[10].

Among recent empirical efforts to assess outcome, at least two major ones should be mentioned. One involves the *Cleveland Health Quality Choice Coalition*, a cooperative instead of the traditional adversary effort among consumer and provider groups aimed at assessing care quality and efficiency at 31 Cleveland hospitals. The coalition was established in 1989 and was at least initially designed to generate comparative outcome data for the hospitals involved. The goal was to implement healthcare purchasing programs which monitored not only costs but also quality. It was patterned after the so called "buy right" healthcare procurement philosophy initially propagated by the Center for Policy Studies in Minneapolis[11]. The underlying rationale was to offer coordinated patient volume incentives to providers in return for demonstrated low cost and high quality care. The former was to be achieved by the cooperation of some 50 large and many more smaller Cleveland-based corporations, while the latter through the comparative but standardized data gathering efforts of the Greater Cleveland Hospital Association, and other organizations representing private physicians[12]. The Coalition was to be managed and essentially run by a 31 member steering committee made up of program participants. All hospitals in the Cleveland area adopted healthcare outcome-based quality measurement systems focusing mainly on patient satisfaction, intensive care as well as medical surgical and obstetrics outcomes - all to be operationally managed and functionally implemented by an organization called the Quality Information Management Corporation (QIMC), a nonprofit entity. It is the QIMC's function through its full-time staff to coordinate hospital data collection efforts, ensure data integrity, and to oversee all operational aspects of the overall project. Patient satisfaction surveys are conducted over three-month patient discharge periods using a random sample of some 600 patients from each participating hospital for each survey cycle. Response rates have varied from 40% to 60%, depending on the hospital. Furthermore, responses are risk adjusted for patient characteristics such as age, sex, education, health insurance, health status, and diagnosis, all beyond the control of the discharging hospital. Intensive care dimensions are assessed in terms of mortality outcomes (quality) and length of stay (efficiency) by comparing expected and outcome data in areas such as admission diagnosis, patient origin (emergency room, other hospital etc.), age, immunological status, and a number of acute physiologic variables (e.g. pulse, neurologic status, blood oxygen, etc.)[13]. In medical, surgical and obstetrical outcome measurement systems, diagnosis specific risk-adjusted models and data were developed to compare inpatient mortality, length of stay, and the occurrence of several negative events among the hospitals. The first comparative hospital report was released in April 1993, with semi-annual reports expected in the future. The initial report included data and information for discharged patients for parts of 1991 and 1992 on intensive care mortality, medical care mortality, length of stay data in most care categories, and patient responses in medical and surgical categories.

The other major empirical quality assessment by way of outcome surveys, concentrating on mortality rates was conducted by the *Department of Veterans Affairs* in VA facilities in 1991[14]. The study was done in two phases. In phase I a statistical analysis using logistic regression models was employed for fourteen different diagnostic categories to patients discharged in 1986 subsequent to having been treated in four different procedure groups (e.g. nonsurgical, therapeutic surgical, diagnostic surgical, other nonoperative but invasive procedures like bronchoscopies). The dependent variable was the patients' health status within 30 days of discharge, while the group of independent variables used included age, race, length of stay, patient origin, admission source, and a number of other variables. Mortality rates were predicted for each medical center taking into account the medical center's patient-mix factors. Quality assessment in terms of outcome was made largely in terms of the ratio of a medical center's observed mortality rate to its predicted rate within specific diagnosis categories, and for entire facilities. Each ratio was viewed in 95% confidence intervals in order to determine if the observed statistics varied more than by chance from expected ones. In phase II, some forty medical centers with unusually elevated mortality rates were singled out for closer scrutiny by medical record peer reviews. Phase I found that twelve of the 172 medical centers examined had overall mortality rates significantly higher than predicted, with observed/predicted ratios ranging from 1.1 to 1.7. Phase II involved some 2,500 cases for some of which no medical records could be found by the time the peer reviews got underway, with ultimately only 577 cases having been referred to a peer review committee pursuant to a screening review. Of those specific cases and their medical records that were peer reviewed, some 20% were found to be inconsistent with current medical practice, with the most frequent problems having centered on unordered or inadequate treatments, missed diagnosis, or unordered diagnostic tests.

Insurance Claims as a Source of Quality Care Data

There have been some proposals to use insurance claims data for attempting to assess care quality, as an alternative or supplement to using individual provider and patient specific information on medical charts[15]. These data are population-based since they focus on beneficiary or enrollee groups, so preventive care, access to any or some care and related issues as well as other healthcare transactions often addressed to entire segments of populations can be examined. The data include information on patient symptoms, diagnoses and diagnostic tests, surgical and other therapeutic procedures, length and intensity of hospitalization, and prescription histories. In addition, claim records can provide information which supplements the usual patient origin data, namely the geographical source of patients, and the demographical characteristics of the patient origin region.

   In addition to their broad scope, data procured from insurance claims may have at least two advantages over raw data generated from patient records, both advantages essentially relating to the cost and facility of procurement. First, procurement and transaction costs incurred for insurance claim data is likely to be much lower than that for patient record. Secondly, primary sourced medical chart data often requires the cooperation of the provider and/or the patient, which is not the case for insurance claim based statistics. Furthermore, within the scope of claim based databases, the so called coding systems, e.g. Current Procedural Terminology - or CPT, used to identify literally thousands of surgical procedures and diagnostic tests can be used for a sophisticated computer based systematic evaluation of provider care and conduct patterns, although very few nondiagnostic and nonsurgical services (counseling, wellness care, etc.) are included in the system[16]. Finally, reimbursements for prescription drug consumption are based on drug types, using the National Drug Code (NDC) categories. Since the codes reflect the exact formulation and strength of the drugs involved and considered for reimbursement, this system may also be used as a source of statistics aimed at care quality assessment. Some unclaimed services, and those covered by deductibles, however, may not be included, making the care data incomplete, particularly regarding those care items which were performed in the initial stages of the encounter with the provider, unless proof that the deductible has been met includes a list of those care items.

Even if claim data did contain a complete inventory of services provided, that would largely address items of care in the care *process* category with little or no explicit information regarding *outcomes*. In this regard, therefore, medical chart abstracts would need to be used to supplement care data extracted from insurance claims in order to define and measure care quality in various instances of implementation. Alternatively, some studies suggested that claim-based data may be used to determine outcome and measure the quality of care if not explicitly then by inference. Thus, a group of hypertensive patients with a given medication may be found to have needed rehospitalization less frequently for hypertensive related ailments than a control group - all of which may be determined from insurance claim-based data[17].

Empirical Patient Surveys and Patient Feedbacks

In standard economic arenas outside of the healthcare sector, a common way to ascertain or at least to intelligently guess what consumers want and like is getting the word from the horse's mouth, the consumers themselves. Various forms of consumer surveys, opinion surveys, "marketing research", and other efforts which keep armies of professionals and paraprofessionals in business are all aimed at trying to produce a product or service which the consumers want, and to find out what consumers think of a product or service once produced and distributed. Consumer feedback in turn governs subsequent management decisions regarding production, quality, design, pricing, distribution, and various other aspects of successfully selling the product or service.

Consumer feedbacks in nonmedical sectors are readily and in general reliably used to assess the technical quality of the product or service, and it is assumed that consumer demand can be favorably diverted by any vendor if it conveys at least the image of a good product at a reasonable price. Similar marketing sentiments are now increasingly viewed as acceptable in health-care markets. However, given the complex nature of the healthcare service, and the sometimes unresolvable labyrinth of complex relationships among the environments, processes and results of healthcare service delivery, the views of the "consumer", the patient, with respect to quality perceptions and other otherwise standard marketing dimensions of healthcare delivery have often been viewed with skepticism. It may be that when it comes to health-care assessment consumers confuse format with substance, quantity with technical quality, and interpersonal relationships with professional com-petence. Thus, it is not surprising that a considerable amount of literature sprung up over the last few years dealing with the pros and cons of asking patients, and relying on their opinion, regarding the quality of their health-care service.

Those that argue against the reliability of consumer surveys do so in general based on the assertion that these surveys reveal more about the con-sumer than about the provider, and that provider personality and charm along with the perceived quantity of the service provided often blurs any technical considerations which the patient may undertake, even if he or she was capable of doing so. Thus, the patient's personal characteristics such as socio-economic status, educational level, age, ethnicity, and others may gross bias even a fundamental tendency to reliably assess physician performance, once again even if the patient was capable of so doing[18]. It is often asserted that consumers can be falsely impressed by the various types and volume of service performed, whether needed or not. High service volume is connoted with conscientious professional performance and technical competence - the more the better when it comes to tests and procedures, some consumers may come to think. Thus, middle-aged patients with chest pain viewed their care better when assigned various but unnecessary tests than those who were not. Or, healthy HMO enrollees found no difference in care quality in comparison to similarly healthy fee-for-service patients in spite of the HMO's tendency to perform less service, but when ill patients were assigned to these two pro-vider groups, fee-for-service patients who received more tests and care service items than HMO patients viewed their care much better than those in HMOs[19]. These are the personal perceptions of the patients. Whether correct or incorrect depends on the relationship between the quantity of tests and care items rendered and the true quality of care. Until that relationship is cleared up, and it may be very difficult to do, there is no way of saying that these consumer perceptions are in fact false, or otherwise.

Reliance on consumer response for technical medical service quality rating is also opposed on the grounds that the consumer is scientifically not sophisticated enough to judge the performance of the physician. Thus, while consumers can judge the physician's personality, at least the personality that is displayed during care service delivery, they cannot judge their technical competence. On the other hand, it is evident that there are considerable variations in consumer sophistication to judge their healthcare provider. Furthermore, there is disagreement even among physicians as to the desired or standard quality of care which was or should have been rendered under given circumstances. If there was none, then, one may argue, there would not exist that substantial number of medical expert witnesses, some of them full-time professionals in that respect, who deliver their opinions in medical malpractice suits contrary to their fellow physicians who are retained on the other side of the same case. At any rate, it was found that when it came to obviously poor quality of care, there appeared to be considerable agreement between patients and providers as to that predicament, which may be important if by some value judgment one considers the identification of poor care socially more desirable than standard or excellent care[20]. In addition, the consumer's ability to assess the technical quality of care is not a constant with respect to the type and sophistication of care rendered, since it was found that for frequently recurring care items quality was correctly perceived[21].

Finally, it is sometimes asserted that patient feedbacks are often clouded by physician personalities. In fact, as to the relationship between patient attitudes and physician personality, there does appear to be a significant correlation. That is, the "nicer" the physician the more technically competent he or she is perceived to be by the patient[22]. The problem is to determine whether the physician's interpersonal skills actually interfere with the patient's ability to objectively assess technical competence. The answer may not be as obvious as it may seem. It is possible that physician congeniality is an integral part of the treatment process and might in fact have a profound impact on the outcome, as we already postulated earlier in the volume. If so, then positively assessed personality is simply an indication of a positively assessable overall healthcare service rendered, and a high correlation between physician personality and positive patient perception is justified. In other words, the physician's interpersonal skills are simply part of his overall technical competence. Only if this was not the case could one assert with some degree of certainty that physician personality in fact interferes with the assessment of technical competence. Furthermore, even this assertion would likely vary with the complexity of the care involved.

Notwithstanding these reservations about using patient feedbacks to assess care quality, there appear to be some serious reasons as well for doing so. In general, these reasons suggest that for better or worse consumer feedbacks may be used to predict consumer behavior, that consumers actually need not be technically qualified to be fair *reporters* of data and information, that consumer feedback data is much cheaper to obtain than possibly other source quality related assessments, it may not be proportionately inferior, and finally whatever consumers opine may not be readily accessible otherwise. It has been found that consumers who are satisfied with their healthcare service recommend it to others, and those that are not simply terminate their relationship with their provider, e.g. disenroll from an HMO. Consumer feedbacks may also be used as simply reported information and could be accurate and valuable when viewed in the context of, or in comparison to, other data and information sources. In other words, consumer reports may be used as controls for other data and information resources, attained at a reasonable cost. In 1987, HCFA calculated that on the average it costs about $55, and a half-hour in terms of time, to procure information from and review a given patient record. Other studies indicated that abstracting medical records according to protocol, a process which in most cases requires the services of skilled nurses, physicians, medical record librarians, and the professional development of algorithms, plus the cost of data entry, averaged about $45 per record. In contrast, it is estimated in general, although it has not been confirmed by systematic studies, that patient surveys tend to cost less. The latter depends on the design and extent of the survey, the length of the questionnaire, mailing, interviewing and follow-up call costs, and so forth[23].

In order to generate patient feedback regarding any quality aspect of care, it is assumed that the patient at least *recalls* important care dimensions, and does so accurately. Some studies attempted to determine the extent and the content of patient recall of the care services rendered to them, and, therefore, the patient's ability to report on some technical or interpersonal aspects of the care in relation to what their medical charts contained. Some studies surveyed recall proportions for various hospitalization experiences, and found that recall for most instances began to wane after about 10 months with events of major financial or medical consequence not surprisingly remembered better than minor ones. Two subsequent studies of ambulatory patients who received care from an HMO found an 88% service utilization recollection after 12 months in comparison with the contents of medical charts[24]. Some research has also been done on specific medication recall but with limited results. In fact, it was mostly found that the recall factor was loose at best, in many cases highly inaccurate, the degree of inaccuracy increasing with the elapsed length of time[25]. Some further studies indicated that diagnostic statements made by physicians during examination are more likely recalled than the advice given by the physician[26].

Many hospitals now routinely seek patient feedback after discharge, however, most of the survey results are not published for a variety of social, economic and political reasons. What survey results have been published deal largely with outpatients. A recently published study attempted to ascertain specific aspects of hospital inpatient care that were perceived by patients as most important to them, and how those perceptions varied by various patient characteristics[27]. The study involved 62 hospitals, while another 80 hospitals also solicited to participate did not partake. The reasons for refusing to participate are interesting as well as perhaps telling of prevailing although no longer necessarily predominant hospital management attitudes towards published care quality related surveys. These reasons included assertions to the effect that there was not enough administrative resources to produce a list of eligible patients in the hospitals, hospital administration simply had no interest in patient reports, inadequate computer systems and data for necessary patient selection, reluctance to reveal hospital identity, internal marketing surveys already underway, unattractiveness of the survey's protocol to the administration, and finally simple refusals by the hospital boards. Less than statistically significant differences were found between participating and non-participating hospitals with a higher frequency of larger and academically affiliated hospitals participating mostly in the Midwest more than in the South.

Some 100 patients from each hospital were surveyed within about three months of their discharge. Some 76% (or about 6,500) of those contacted responded to telephone surveys while the rest simply refused or said they were too sick to participate. The interviews were scored by the proportion of negative responses received in each surveyed care service area. An average of scores for each area constituted the summary score. Although different care areas were surveyed with different intensity and with different numbers of questions, no weighting was deemed necessary to account for these differences.

The main problem areas perceived across all patient characteristics appear to be related to patient-doctor communications. In particular, almost half of those surveyed complained about not being told what their daily routine should be, almost as many complained of not being told whom to contact for future help, and some 25% felt a lack of physician availability to answer questions. In addition, a significant number of those surveyed felt that they were not adequately advised as to the pain or discomfort to expect, and in general did not receive understandable answers from physicians and nurses, and a relatively small proportion complained of a lack of privacy when being advised of their conditions, or that their condition should have been conveyed without upsetting them. Between 10% and 20% of the patients surveyed in those categories perceived problems in their relationship with hospital staff, such as not knowing the amount of moneys they will owe, or how to pay, general patient needs were not met, several service omissions, and lack of patient involvement in care decisions. In the emotional support category, almost 40% of those surveyed perceived a lack of mutual trust with anyone in the hospital except with the physician in charge of the case. The survey included a variety of other categories such as physical comfort, pain management, education, family involvement, and preparation for discharge and future care. Some 30% felt that nurses were overworked and gave inadequate care, 25%-30% felt that important side effects of medicines were not clearly conveyed, and 20%-30% felt that in general they were ill-prepared to leave the hospital by not being alerted to danger signals to look out for, or told what to and what not to eat, and what to and what not to do so as not to endanger their condition. In terms of patient characteristics, younger patient groups appeared to be slightly more critical than older ones, females more than males, less educated ones very slightly more than educated ones, poorer people more than wealthy ones, those in non-white race categories more than whites, and, significantly but perhaps not surprising and with possibly limited usefulness for care quality assessment, those in poor health after discharge almost twice as unhappy as those in excellent health.

The main sources for problem perceptions appear to center on post discharge health status and socio-economic, and based on the regression results these two factors appear to be the strongest predictors for problem perceptions even if other factors such as race, insurance status, length-of-stay, and other medically specific factors were taken into consideration. Notwithstanding the above, the regression model involving these noted variables accounted for only 9% of the variance in the problem score, indicating that other factors such as institutional characteristics, general hospital administrative policy, other care conditions specific to the hospital or to the patient unaccounted for by the model must also play an important role. This study is notable in several respects. First, as limited as its scope is within the context of the national hospital environment because of the relatively limited number of institutions participating, it appears to be the first published national hospital survey of patient perceptions shortly after discharge. When viewed in terms of the traditional structure-process-outcome models, the study may be viewed as somewhat structure oriented, heavily relying on process variables, and including some outcome dimensions, such as health status. However, health status (an outcome variable) was shown to be a relatively major determinant of problem perceptions with the latter having been expressed in process and structure dimensions, and that creates a circulatory logic when one attempts to use this model for some sort of care quality assessment. In other words, perceived outcome reflected and reacted upon perceived process and structure rendering care quality assessment in terms of the traditional (Donabedian) logical model essentially indeterminate. If a patient was feeling well within the surveyed three month post-discharge period chances are that he or she reflected upon inpatient experiences less unfavorably than if that patient was feeling ill. Thus, apart from the fact that true care outcome in this study is quite blurred and may even be unknown because it is based on a short three-month post discharge period during which the true or ultimate outcome of care may not be known or evident to anyone including the patient, this outcome was found to have a profound but nonetheless superficial effect on structure and process perceptions. Because of this, it would be impossible to ascertain from the study whether or not the quality of care was good or up to standard, for poor health status can result from excellent care, and seemingly very good but likely temporary health status can result from quite substandard care, each yielding their corresponding positive or negative perceptions within the context of the structure and process factors utilized in the study. In fact, this reservation may be asserted about most consumer surveys aimed at rigorously assessing care quality, thus relegating these surveys to secondary roles in concerted efforts to assess care quality, and only supplemental to traditional medical record-based and protocol-controlled assessments. In a supplemental role these surveys can be very useful for, as we pointed out earlier, they provide relatively low cost information and data not available from other sources, and ascertaining whether or not patient expectations have been met in terms of the dispensed care, particularly in terms of the various dimensions of the all important physician-patient communication, may also be an essential variable in the overall healthcare quality equation. In addition, it is hard to match the completeness of a study based on medical records. All discharged patients' quality controlled records are there for examination. Consumer surveys on the one hand are voluntary, often very incomplete, and likely to be personally biased. Many hospitals do not wish to be surveyed, particularly if the survey results are published. Even if acceding to a survey, hospitals may be selective in terms of making patient contact points available, allowing access to some patients and not to others. In view of these and several other easily postulated problems, survey results are likely to be positively biased, leaving a host of existing problems relating healthcare quality simply unrevealed.

The Impact of the Healthcare System

Questions have often been raised and answers often postulated if the US style healthcare system, in contrast to those more government based and controlled as in other countries such as Canada, Germany, Japan and elsewhere, generates better quality of care[28]. A most recent study, comparing the Canadian and US systems, appears to provide an answer in the affirmative. It is significant as some healthcare policy analysts appear to prefer the Canadian system to that of the US, particularly in view of its inherent controls on utilization and, therefore, presumably on costs. For instance, in the area of cardiac care, a major concern for predominant population segments beyond a certain age in both countries whether patients in the US are more likely to experience procedures such as cardiac catherization, balloon agioplasty, or coronary artery bypass graft surgery than those in Canada. Clearly, a negative cost indicator for the US, but is it a negative quality indicator? The evidence presented in a recent study appears to point to the contrary[29]. The database for this study contained some 41,000 heart-attack patients from a prior international study conducted between 1990 and 1993 in which different strategies were used to test the efficacy of so called cardiac artery "clotbusters". All patients used in this 1994 study, randomly selected from the prior 1990-93 study, received these cardiac artery clotbusters. These patients were asked to account for the quality of their life during three alternative time periods after discharge: 30 days, six months, and one year. It was found that Canadian patients remained hospitalized about one day longer than their US counterparts, although they went through less cardiac procedures than US patients. Some 80% of the US patients were hospitalized at institutions with cardiac catheterization facilities compared with 38% in Canada, reflecting perhaps on the greater number of cardiologists in the US than in Canada. While inpatients, only 25% of the Canadians went through coronary angiography compared to 72% in the US. Similarly, with respect to angioplasty and coronary bypass surgeries the US-Canadian comparative rates were 29%-11% and 14%-3% respectively. By the end of the one year period, only 24% of the Canadians in comparison to 53% of the US patients were subjected to coronary angioplasty or bypass surgery at least once. How did US patients feel emotionally and physically in comparison to Canadian ones at the end of the first year? Responses to a survey suggested that patients in the US were better off than those in Canada, perhaps because of the more intensive care utilization. When comparing physical capacities before and after the heart attacks, 22% found them worse in the US versus 35% in Canada. Work habits and ability to perform at their occupations were changed for 57% of the Canadians while only for 37% of the US patients. Shortness of breath and chest pain encounters between US and Canadian patients were 29% vs. 45% and 21% vs. 34%, respectively. US patients, having experienced greater degrees of care and facility utilization, also experienced a better health status at least during the first year after their heart attack. In general, the outcomes in the US were better than in Canada. However, these results should be assessed in view of the fact that in the two countries essentially two different care practices and medications were implemented with respect to these patients, and that in the US the patients have more likely encountered a specialist than in Canada. However, the study does appear to cast doubt on frequent concerns that greater resource utilization in the US does not generate improved outcome here, that is, it does not incrementally benefit the patients, although it markedly increases healthcare costs. The question whether a relatively modest outcome advantage in the US warrants a substantially greater degree of resource utilization is another one for health economists, healthcare policy analysts and policy makers, healthcare ethicists, and last but certainly not least for providers.

Notes

1.   Leape, L.L., Lawthers, A.G., Brennan, T.A., Johnson, W.G., "Preventing Medical Injury", *QRB*, May 1993, citing Brennan, T.A. et al., "Incidence of Adverse Events

and Negligence in Hospitalized Patients: Results from the Harvard Medical Practice Study I", *New England Journal of Medicine,* Vol. 324, 1991, and Leape, L.L. et al., "The Nature of Adverse Events in Hospitalized Patients: Results from the Harvard Medical Practice Study II", *New England Journal of Medicine,* Vol. 324, 1991.

2.   Leape, L.L. et al., 1993, pp. 146-47.

3.   Health Care Financing Administration, *The Uniform Clinical Data Set System,* HCFA, Health Care Standards and Quality Bureau, Office of Peer Review, Division of Program Assessment and Information, Baltimore, MD.

4.   Hartz, A.J., Sigmann, P., Guse, C., Hagen, T.C., "The System of the Uniform Clinical Data Set System (UCDSS) in a Hospital Setting", *The Joint Commission Journal on Quality Improvement,* March 1994.

5.   Health Care Financing Administration, *MQIS/CCP Project Newsletter,* No. 4, July 1994.

6.   Donaldson, M.S., "Gearing Up for Health Data in the Information Age", *The Joint Commission Journal on Quality Improvement,* April 1994.

7.   Knaus, W.A., Draper, E.A., Wagner, D.P. and Zimmerman, J.E., "Prognosis in Acute System Failure", *Annals of Surgery,* Vol. 202, 1985. See also Wagner, D.P., Knaus, W.A. and Draper, E.A., "Physiologic Abnormalities and Outcome from Acute Disease", *Archives of Internal Medicine,* Vol. 146, 1986.

8.   Hadorn, D., Baker, D., Dracup, K., Pitt, B., "Making Judgements About Treatment Effectiveness Based on Health Outcomes: Theoretical and Practical Issues", *Joint Commission Journal on Quality Improvement,* October 1994.

9.   Iezzoni, L.I., Greenber, L.G., "Widespread Assessment of Risk-Adjusted Outcomes: Lessons From Local Initiative", *Joint Commission Journal on Quality Improvement,* June 1994. See also, Iezzoni, L.I., "Risk Adjustment for Medical Outcomes Studies" in Grady, M.I. (ed.), *Medical Effectiveness Research Data Methods,* Agency for Healthcare Policy and Research, Rockville, MD, 1992; Iezzoni, L.I., *Risk Adjustment for Measuring Healthcare Outcomes,* Health Administration Press, Ann Arbor, MI, 1994; and Iezzoni, L.I., Schwartz, M., Restuccia, J.D., "The Role of Severity Information in Health Policy Debates: A Survey of State and Regional Concerns", *Inquiry,* Vol. 28, Summer 1991.

10.   Refer to discussions earlier in this volume regarding the value and reliability for care quality evaluations of published mortality statistics for various hospitals. See also Park, R.E. et. al., "Explaining Variations in Hospital Death Rates, Randomness, Severity of Illness, Quality of Care", *JAMA,* Vol. 264, 1990; Fink, A., Yano, E.M., Brook, R.H., "The Condition of the Literature on Differences in Hospital Mortality", *Medical Care,* Vol. 27, 1989; Thomas, J.W., Holloway, J.J., Guire, K.E., "Validating Risk-Adjusted Mortality as an Indicator for Quality of Care", *Inquiry,* Vol. 30, 1993.

11.   Iglehart, J.K., "Competition and the Pursuit of Quality: A Conversation With Walter McClure", *Health Affairs,* Vol. 7, Spring 1988. See also Winslow, R., "Data Spur Debate on Hospital Quality", *Wall Street Journal,* May 24, 1990; and, Ellwood, P.M., "Shattuck Lecture - Outcomes Management: A Technology of Patient Management", *New England Journal of Medicine,* 1988.

12.   The Greater Cleveland Hospital Association has as its members some 60 Northeastern Ohio hospitals. The organization representing the interests of some 3,000 private physicians was the Academy of Medicine of Cleveland. Corporations were pulled together through "Cleveland Tomorrow", a chamber of commerce type of corporate excecutive sponsored establishement, and by the Health Council of Northeast Ohio, a corporate employment and employee benefit executive body. Group health purchasing efforts on the part of smaller businesses were represented by the Council

of Smaller Enterprises with about 13,000 members. See Shaller, D.V., Woods, P., "Reforming the Market for Value in Healthcare: The Cleveland Experience", *Journal of Occupational Medicine,* Vol. 35, 1991; Sadler, J., "Small Business Fears Long-term Effects of Health Plan", *Wall Street Journal,* Oct 4, 1993

13. Sirio, C.A. et al., "Evaluation of Hospital Performance in Metropolitan Hospital ICUs: The Cleveland Health Quality Choice Project (CHQCP), *Clinical Research,* Vol. 41, 1993; Knaus, W.A. et al., "APACHE - Acute Physiology and Chronic Health Evaluation: A Physiologically Based Classification System, *Critical Care Medicine,* Vol. 9, 1981.

14. Department of Veterans Affairs, *Review of Mortality in VA Medical Centers,* Washington, DC, 1989; and Department of Veterans Affairs, *Supplement to Review of Mortality in VA Medical Centers,* Washington, DC, 1992.

15. Lohr, K.N., "Use of Insurance Claims Data in Measuring Quality of Care", *International Journal of Technology Assessment in Health Care,* Vol. 6, 1990; and Steinberg, E.P., Whittle, J. and Anderson, G.F., "Impact of Claims Data Research on Clinical Practice", *International Journal of Technology Assessment in Health Care,* Vol. 6, 1990.

16. Luft, H.S., Hunt, S.S., "Evaluating Individual Hospital Quality Through Outcomes Statistics", *JAMA,* Vol. 255, 1986. See also Lohr, K.N. and Schroeader, S.A., "Strategy for Quality Assurance in Medicare", *New England Journal of Medicine,* Vol. 332, 1990. See also Brook, R.H., Williams, K.N., Rolph, J.E., "Controlling the Use and Cost of Medical Services: The New Mexico Experimental Medical Care Review Organization - A Four Year Study", *Medical Care* (Supplement), Vol. 16, 1978. The CPT codes have been used to evaluate the propriety of antibiotic injections administered by Medicare providers.

17. See Maronde, R.F. et al., "Underutilization of Antihypertensive Drugs and Associated Hospitalization", *Medical Care,* Vol. 27, 1989.

18. Ware, J.E., Davies-Avery, A., Stewart, A.L., "The Measurement and Meaning of Patient Satisfaction", *Health and Medical Care Services Review,* Vol. 1, 1978, and Linn, L.S. and Greenfield, S., "Patient Suffering and Patient Satisfaction", *Medical Care,* Vol. 22, 1984. See also Lebow, J.L., "Consumer Assessment of the Quality of Medical Care", *Medical Care,* Vol. 12, 1974; Linn, L.S., "Factors Associated With Patient Evaluation of Healthcare", *Milbank Memorial Fund Quarterly,* Vol. 53, 1975; Linder-Peltz, S., "Social Psychological Determinants of Patient Satisfacion: A Test of Five Hypotheses", *Social Science and Medicine,* Vol. 15, 1982.

19. Sox, H.C. Jr., Margulies, I. and Sox, C.H., "Psychologically Mediated Effects of Diagnostic Tests", *Annals of Internal Medicine,* Vol. 95, 1981; Davies, A.R., "Consumer Acceptance of PrePaid and Fee-for-Service Care: Results from a Randomized Trial", *Health Services Research,* Vol. 21, 1986.

20. Ehrlich, J., Morehead, M.A., Trussell, R.E., *The Quantity, Quality and Cost of Medical and Hospital Care Secured by a Sample of Teamster Families in the New York Area,* Columbia University School of Public Health and Administrative Medicine, New York, 1961.

21. Ware, J.E., Snyder, M.K., Wright, W.R., *Development and Validation of Scales to Measure Patient Satisfaction with Healthcare Services.* Vol. I. Part B: *Results Regarding Scales Constructed from the Patient Satisfaction Questionnaire and Measures of Other Health Perceptions,* National Technical Information Service, Springfield VA, 1976; and Hulka, B.S. et al., "Scale for the Measurement of Attitudes Towards Physicians and Primary Medical Care", *Medical Care,* Vol. 8, 1970.

22. See note 21.

23. Davies, A.R., Ware, J.E. Jr., "Involving Consumers in Quality of Care Assessment", *Health Affairs*, Spring 1988.
24. National Center for Health Statistics, *Reporting of Hospitalization in the Health Interview Survey*, Vital and Health Statistics Series 2, No. 6 USGPO, Washington, DC, 1965; National Center for Health Statistics, Health Interview Responses Compared with Medical Records, Vital and Health Statistics Series 2, No. 7, USGPO, Washington, DC, 1966; National Center for Health Statistics, *Net Differences in Interview Data on Chronic Conditions and Information Derived From Medical Records*. Vital and Health Statistics Series 2, No. 57 DHEW Publ. HSM 73-1331 June 1973, USGPO, Washington, DC, 1973; Harlow, S.D. and Linet, M.S., "Agreement Between Questionnaire Data and Medical Records: The Evidence for Accuracy of Recall", *American Journal of Epidemiology*, Vol. 129, 1989.
25. Paganini-Hill, A., Ross, R.K., "Reliability of Recall of Drug Usage and Other Health Related Information", *American Journal of Epidemiology*, Vol. 116, 1982; Hulka, B.S., Kupper, L.L., Cassel, J.C., Efird, R.L., "Medication Use Misuse: Physician-Patient Discrepancies", *Journal of Chronic Diseases*, Vol. 28, 1975. See also Gerbert, B., Stone, G. et al., "Agreement Among Physician Assessment Methods: Searching for the Truth Among Fallible Methods", *Medical Care*, Vol. 26, 1988.
26. Schraa, J.S., Dirks, J.F., "Improving Patient Recall and Comprehension of the Treatment Regimen", *Journal of Asthma*, Vol. 1982; Ley, P., Spelman, M.S., "Communications in an Outpatient Setting", *British Journal of Clinical Psychology*, Vol. 4, 1965; and, Page, D., Verstraet, D.G., Robb. J.R., Etzwiler, D.D., "Patient Recall of Self-Care Recommendations in Diabetes", *Diabetes Care*, Vol. 4, 1981. For a more recent recall study of various diagnostic and therapeutic procedures in ambulatory settings, also refer to Brown, J.B. and Adams, M.E., "Patients as Reliable Reporters of Medical Care Process: Recall of Ambulatory Encounter Events", *Medical Care*, Vol. 30, No. 5, 1992.
27. Cleary, P.D., Edgeman-Levitan, S., Roberts, M., Moloney, T.W. et al., "Patients Evaluate Their Hospital Care: A National Survey", Data Watch, *Health Affairs*, Winter 1991.
28. See Seplaki, L., *Cost and Competition in American Medicine*, University Press of America, Lanham, MD, 1994, Chs 26-28.
29. Mark, D.B., Naylor, C.D., Hlatky, M.A. et al., "Use of Medical Resources and Quality of Life After Acute Myocardial Infarction in the US and Canada", *New England Journal of Medicine*, October 27, 1994, pp. 1130-1135.

6 Institutional Healthcare Quality

Historically, hospitals have been competing in terms of technology and quality, but rarely price because the latter was, for various legal and professional reasons, generally excluded from selective contracting. The presence of and application to diagnostics and treatment of high level medical structure by way of sophisticated technology *presupposed* superior care process and generally desirable outcomes, without effective measurement efforts. In recent years, hospital care service purchase decision processes by private and public consumer groups have often utilized price, cost consciousness pervaded the medical scene, and quality constraints in terms of widely disseminated process and outcome standards, both prescribed and attained, are now an integral part of hospital service transactions. Thus, hospital competitive variables include price, and various measurable and measured dimensions of care quality simultaneously. Economic theory, traditionally formulated to analyze and predict rational economic behavior in nonmedical markets, can now be relatively readily applied to medical markets, if purchasers are aware of and understand the various price and quality dimensions in terms of which hospitals are now compelled to compete. In fact, even if there is some lack of information and price flexibility, that is, if product quality cannot be ascertained in advance of purchase, some elements of insurance can abridge the gap.

Classical economic theories of market behavior assign complete knowledge and information to the consumer on the quality of products purchased. Relative price levels suggest relatively recognized qualities, and consumers make their choices based on those variables. Price fluctuations allow market responses to consumer choices until such time as the market clears its inventory of all quality level products and services sold at their respective price levels. All products and services, whether high or low in quality and, therefore, whether high or low in price will be sold. Prices are seen to reflect product or service quality and are considered as the overall market barometer. If the consumer is uncertain about product quality in spite of the presence of relative prices, then suppliers rely on nonprice, indirect market "signaling" of quality to consumers, as well as on rationing[1].

Failure of consumers to ascertain product or service quality can also set off a "desupply spiral". If there are major quality differences, but consumers cannot assess or appreciate these differences hence are unwilling to pay a higher than average price for better than average products, the latter will not be supplied causing a reduction in the general (average) quality level of supplied products and, consequently, the prices which consumers are willing to pay. Original average product costs will no longer be covered by the prices consumers pay, hence those will not be produced either. The spiral will continue until supply dwindles down to zero - a natural reaction to a lack of information and understanding of product quality on the part of the consumers and a natural consequence of what appears to be a rational behavior on the part of the suppliers. The so called "market signaling" has been seen to overcome this predicament. Thus, employers may judge the quality of their potential employees' (the suppliers/sellers of their own labor) contribution to their business on the basis the employees' attained education, and the employees attempt to "signal" that contribution by adequately preparing themselves for the labor market in terms of their educational attainment. Or, producers may want to "signal" the quality of their product by allowing consumers to "experience" the product (purchase it) at a price initially lower than what they would normally want to receive for it to cover the cost or to generate some preconceived profit margin, and subsequently raise the price after allowing consumers to experience the quality of the product involved and time for an increase and establishment of the product's reputation. It is further assumed that the "post-experience" price will be high enough not only to generate expected profits but also to recoup the possible losses caused by the initially low "experience price levels"[2].

Medical market choices by consumers and responses by medical service suppliers begin to approximate traditional and more recent modern economic reasoning and market choices based on the price-quality dichotomy due to the emerging importance of quality assessment more in terms of process and particularly outcome than by way of traditional structural considerations alluded to earlier. In the past, inter-hospital competition was predicated upon the technology utilized and the formal qualifications of the staff affiliated with the hospital. As we noted in the earlier parts of the volume, these attributes however do not necessarily and even causally assure desirable care processes or outcomes. Furthermore, because of inter-hospital competitive pressures, capital facilities, sophisticated diagnostic and therapeutic equipment have until very recently been widely duplicated in a number of major hospitals and medical centers in the same region, with hospitals attempting to secure their share of regional image and reputation in relation to those of their competitors. These structural attributes, even if they were reliable yardsticks of process and outcome quality, could no longer single out the best hospital(s) in any given market. Even more recently, with the intensification of cost containment efforts and related pressures by large and coordinated healthcare service buyers, hospitals in many community/regional markets began to share large, expensive and sophisticated equipment and similar facilities, leaving the exclusive possession, if not use, of those facilities only to major university affiliated medical centers. Thus, these structural attributes diminish in their significance as care quality indicators.

Consequently, quality concerns have been refocused upon care processes and outcomes. As we noted earlier, data are being cultivated and analyzed relating to procedure specific outcomes such as death rates, readmissions, and complications. Subsequent to patient discharge from hospitals, medical chart data are abstracted by specialized services into various datasets and data bases, the use of peer review organizations for Medicare patients, for the utilization of healthcare research and health policy scholars, and for the scrutiny of health agencies in many of the states. Hospital specific favorable conclusions drawn from this type of data are increasingly used by hospitals in their competitive marketing efforts. Thus, hospital market environments are beginning to approximate market conditions long envisioned by economists for non-medical products and services where customers of all type can choose from various well-understood care options with explicit quality and price levels. Structural buildups with their associated waste and excessive costs, become redundant as customer choice is based on process/outcome specific quality and price. The availability of reliable and consumer understood quality information enables price competition, while a lack of those variables renders price competition impotent, or outright impossible. Much of this is to be understood in the light of the various qualifications and caveats, which have been extensively covered earlier, in particular that much of the outcome data need to be risk-adjusted and weighted in terms of the particulars of the hospital's case-mix. This latter consideration may lead to the possibility that in order to control outcome, hospitals may attempt to control their admitted case-mix, more so when we consider the impact of the Medicare DRG payment system's similar predisposition to and contingency upon case-mixes, as some diagnoses receive higher reimbursements than others. The logical economic answer on the part of the hospitals is nonprice rationing of services, a practice that has long been in place with insurance companies who, for instance, may deny certain coverage for pre-existing conditions. Thus, hospitals may implement nonprice rationing by simply not equipping themselves to care for high-risk patients, by carefully selecting the services they offer or by choosing those medical staff affiliates who are less likely to deliver high-risk patients.

Hospital Performance: Dimensions and Measurements

During the past few years much progress has been attained in quality assessment, in particular quality assurance by way of outcome evaluation. Quality signals such as unanticipated readmissions and inpatient mortality have become centers of attention. Various hospital attributes and care quality dimensions were correlated for the purpose of predicting care quality. Thus, standardized mortality rates were used to reflect on possible higher care quality in not for-profit institutions than in for-profit ones and in community institutions. Studies of this type may assist third-party payers, including the government and insurers, to make economically rational purchasing decisions in increasingly competitive healthcare markets[3]. Mortality rate differentials, however, can be a source for unfair even libelous judgments and quality assessments. It has been argued for instance that HCFA's methods for quality assessment based on mortality rates do not adequately allow for differences in the nature and severity in patient illness. Thus, acute care centers which typically care for more severely ill patients are also more likely to have higher mortality rates, notwithstanding the fact that they may be well managed administratively and clinically. In addition, mortality rate differences may also be due to random variations among institutions unrelated to the quality of care[4].

Given the shortcomings of relative mortality rates as measures of hospital care quality, alternative means of hospital care quality assessments have been experimented with. Measurements based on adverse events and negligence were advanced, with the alleged advantage that they are derived from a careful review of medical records and charts, instead of administrative records. Medical records in general contain much more information than discharge forms or claims, yet the latter seem to be used more often for readmission and mortality rate studies. In addition, it has been argued that using adverse events rather than morbidity or mortality statistics reflects on medical management in the process phase of the care not the evolution of the patient's disease process itself[5]. However, to the extent that many adverse events may in fact be unavoidable and unpredictable, and that these events themselves may be affected or even brought about by the severity of the illness itself or the complexity of the care applied, adverse events may be plagued with the same maladies as yardsticks of care quality as are mortality rates or re-admissions. It has often been found that surgical specialities and institutions largely caring for acutely ill individuals have higher rates of adverse events than other institutional providers. Nevertheless, if adverse events can be clearly associated with negligence instead of being an unavoidable by-product of illness severity, they can be viewed as an indicator of care quality. A relatively recent study appears to have sorted some of these issues out. It used a sample of 31,000 medical records from 51 randomly selected hospitals in New York State. It found significant variations in adverse event rates among institutions and adverse event rates that could be attributed to negligence. Thus, adverse event rates in general were found to be higher in primary teaching institutions than in rural community hospitals. However, this may be due to the higher frequency of acutely ill patients treated in primary teaching institutions and also to the higher frequency if invasive treatments procedures applied. In fact, this appears to be confirmed by findings to the effect that when it came to adverse events caused by negligence, primary teaching and for-profit hospitals fared significantly better than rural community not for-profit hospitals and institutions that cared mainly for minority patients. Adverse events in general and negligence caused adverse events which were found not to be randomly distributed and could be viewed as indicators of substandard care patterns with certain types of institution[6].

Another relatively recent study attempted to construct three risk adjusted indices of hospital performance from discharge abstracts for mortality, readmissions and complications[7]. While it would be more appropriate to rate hospital care quality directly by measuring *changes* in the patients' health status pursuant to treatment in the hospital, that type of comparative study would require health status data regarding the patients prior and subsequent to hospitalization, a data gathering task that would be difficult to implement for hundreds of thousands of patients and a large national hospital sample. The three indices are to proxy relative patient outcomes, and the quality of care at each hospital is assumed to vary inversely with the rates of these adverse events, that is, a higher quality of care service is presumed with lower rates of these three categories of adverse events. In order to construct these indices, two related problems had to be accounted for: case-mix and case complexity differences among hospitals, to eliminate risk biases in favor of hospitals that treat patients with less complexity or severity. In this connection, the so called "indirect standardization" methods classify diseases into categories of homogeneous elements with similar risks and outcome predictions. Medicare's Prospective Payment (DRG) classification system for hospitals may serve a purpose such as that, so that within each DRG further classification can be made based on risks[8]. To calculate risk factor the study utilized some six million discharge abstracts from the national all-payer datafile of the Commission on Professional and Hospital Activities (CPHA's). The indices estimate the differences in the reasons for admission among the patients treated in various hospitals, leaving the estimation of hospital performance differentials as residuals.

A 1992 study essentially extended this idea by way of a derivative issue. Can changes in the severity of inpatient illnesses be interpreted as some sort of measures of hospital performance[9]. The study hypothesized that, in general, hospital inpatient care varied directly with the patient's condition while hospitalized. Severity was measured by a so called Consumer Severity Index (CSI) using the MedisGroups method. CSI abstracts disease-specific data from medical records and ranks severity on a scale from 1 to 4, where the initial level of severity is based on the patient's condition over a 24 hour period from the time of admission, and the maximum severity represent the worst condition over the entire period of hospitalization (e.g. if death occurs, that would represent a score of 4, otherwise the most severe condition short of death). MedisGroup rates admission severity from 0 to 4 based on clinical information abstracted from medical records also covering the first 24 hour post-admission condition of the patient, plus a "midstay" period extending from the third to the seventh day of hospital stay. The study included 233 patients with myocardial infarction and 279 coronary artery by-pass graft patients in four New England hospitals in 1987. It found that acute myocardial infraction patients who worsened had more potential quality problems than the other patients in the study, specifically under CSI some 71% of the patients with worsening condition experienced care quality problems, with similar results under MedisGroup essentially confirming this predicament. The results for coronary artery bypass grafts were also in the same range of numbers. After death-related data was removed from the study, patient condition patterns ("clinical trajectory") continued to point to care quality problems, further suggesting a positive correlation between worsening (but survived) condition and substandard care quality. The study clearly points to the possibility that the worsening condition (increasing "illness severity") of patients in hospital settings may be indicative of substandard care, depending on the patient's condition, measurement of severity, and the definition of care quality standards and problems.

What about early *re*-admission specifically as an inpatient care quality indicator? Undue early re-admission could be viewed as a care quality problem or as an adverse outcome, under some circumstances. However, some equalization of related factors need to be achieved so as to use this occurrence as a care quality yardstick. Thus, it needs to be ascertained whether certain types of cases (or DRG categories) and case severity levels within each of those DRG categories are more likely to beget early re-admission than others, hence the re-admission differences may not be viewed as an indicator of quality differences. Do hospital size and other care institutional characteristics determine or impact early re-admissions? How about the length-of-stay, a concern quite topical due to the constrained length of hospitalization under the Medicare Prospective Payment (DRG) system. Also, it may be that patients discharged into their home environments are more likely to be readmitted early than those discharged into some sort of professional care or institutional environment. Finally, what does *early* re-admission mean in the first place? What is "early", what is "normal", and what may be "late" re-admission into an acute care environment? Clearly, some sort of time frame needs to be established, and it may that late re-admission pursuant to the physicians' judgment at the hospital is as much of a quality indicator as early re-admission would be. One study used a 31-day period after the last discharge to establish early re-admission[10]. In addition, even if re-admission occurs, it needs to be determined whether such re-admission was unpredicted or unpredictable, or was it a part of a pre-planned regimen of care for the patient. It is obviously easier to ask questions and postulate likely problems than to arrive at answers. These are difficult questions and complex problems, and much research as well as many elaborate empirical studies will need to be conducted to determine some *reliable* framework for using early re-admission as an institutional inpatient care quality indicator.

Some Economic Determinants of Hospital Care Quality

To identify "determinants" of hospital care quality in an exhaustive manner would be a very difficult task, particularly in the light of the problems involved in defining and measuring care quality in the first place, as we just saw. In other words, if we have problems defining and measuring care quality, how do we know what factors determine it and particularly how they determine it? If we have problems identifying the entity how can we study those factors that act upon it? These realistic as well as rhetorical questions are designed more to alert the reader to the issues and problems involved than to discourage an earnest researcher from making some attempts at resolving them.

If we assume some valid definitions of and measurement methods for institutional care quality, as we discussed earlier in this volume, then we may examine some factors which can be viewed in some direct or indirect economic relationship to various notions of care quality and efficiency. For instance, new medical graduates have long represented a source of cheap labor for teaching hospitals. Yet, questions have been raised for some time as to whether or not the lack of experience of this *new staff* contributes negatively to healthcare quality and efficiency, especially during their early months of practical training. In general, some studies have noted that teaching hospitals are more expensive than those not affiliated with medical schools. Additional per case costs at teaching hospitals ranged from about 10% to 30%, compared to other hospitals, notwithstanding, and adjusting for, the fact that patients in teaching hospitals generally require more complex and elaborate care and procedure items, and probably due in large measure to the increased volume of services dispensed at these institutions[11]. It has also been suggested, as well as contradicted, that inexperienced house staff may often generate longer hospital stays, and order more tests and supplies[12]. As to the impact of experience on care quality, one can readily speculate that increased experience improves clinical judgment and technical skill, although past research does not seem to be consistent in this regard. While it has been found by some that teaching hospitals do provide better quality of care, patients often express concern about the quality of care received from residents. Clinical expertise was found to increase with experience, yet no consistent quality deterioration was found in connection with the services performed by residents in many clinical or care environments[13]. A recent study using some 21,000 hospital discharge data looked at both the efficiency and quality implications of training new physicians at teaching hospitals. Measures of efficiency included length of stay and total hospital charges, while measures of quality were hospital deaths, early re-admissions, and nursing home placements. It found that per discharge length of stay and patient cost varied inversely with the staff experience, but found no significant relationship between staff experience and the quality indicators of hospital deaths, re-admissions or nursing home placements[14].

An economic factor which may directly impact on hospital care quality is the hospital's *financial profile*. This becomes increasingly important as competition in hospital markets gains further momentum, and some hospitals may resort to various cost-cutting measures, including some truncated dimensions of quality, to survive. There does not appear to be a wealth of information on the relationship between hospital care quality and the institution's financial profile. However, an inverse relationship was observed between the cost of hospital payroll per bed on the one hand and adjusted mortality rates as well as peer review noted adversities on the other[15]. The treated patients' financial resources directly impact on the hospital's financial profile which may, in turn, affect the quality of care. This was recognized by the federal government through special subsidy provisions for inner-city hospitals in poor neighborhoods that service indigent and largely uninsured patients. These areas usually generate high healthcare cost provoking patient population with minimum or no financial resources of their own for healthcare, including their Medicaid coverage, hence causing these hospitals to be financial losers. Although the HCFA's prospective payment reimbursements to these hospitals contain special adjustments to cover their revenue gap and to encourage them to provide at least standard minimum care, in terms of quantity and quality, to their patient population there are questions as to whether or not these institutions break even and if they do in fact provide adequate care to their patients[16].

One study a couple of years ago directly addressed this issue. Specifically, it sought to determine if there was a relationship between hospital patients' socioeconomic status and the occurrence frequency of medical negligence or substandard service prompted adverse events[17]. Some 50 New York State hospitals were involved and from over 30,000 medical records from 1984 data on medical injury and substandard care were abstracted by gender, race, payer status, and patient income. A strong and inverse relationship was found between payer status and the incidence of substandard care caused medical injuries. Given controlled patient race, income, and gender variables, those without insurance are twice as likely to be victims of negligent care than those with adequate insurance, suggesting a lack of adequate insurance as the main socioeconomic culprit for inadequate care quality. The reasons suggested for this predicament may rest with the uninsured's inability to get proper preventive or diagnostic ambulatory care in the first place, thus forcing them to seek out care in emergency clinics where the normally faster pace of diagnostic and treatment procedures may compromise care quality more than those experienced in other environments.

Hospitals may encounter financial difficulties for a variety reasons. These, in addition to internal management problems and operating inefficiencies, include uncompensated care, withheld or delayed government reimbursements, inability to attracted well-insured patients, high HIV or TB patient population, the predominance of part-time nursing and inadequately qualified physician staffing, and market conditions such as intense competition among a number of hospitals with excess capacity. A more recent, related to the one mentioned earlier, study undertook to determine if there was a relationship between hospital financial profiles and the incidence of negligence caused adverse events. The same 30,000+ medical records from 51 New York State acute care hospitals in 1984 were used to generate financial status, hospital staffing, and adverse events related data. The likelihood of negligence caused medical injury was found to vary inversely with inpatient operating costs per discharge, and a large proportion of the lowest inpatient operating costs were found in financially distressed hospitals serving indigent patient populations[18].

Hospital Mortality Rates Revisited

Easily obtainable administrative data, such as name, age, gender, diagnosis and last hospitalization, can readily be used to locate institutional providers where people die, or die more often than at other hospitals. That information, however, may or may not be a reliable indicator of the relative or absolute care quality provided by these institutions. Hospitals associated with higher death rates do not necessarily offer inferior service. This may not have always been clear to healthcare policy makers and even to the HCFA. Since 1986, the latter has been releasing hospital-specific mortality data and relevant analyses for Medicare patients presumably in the hope that if such data is adequately treated and analyzed it will somehow identify institutions that provide substandard care. In fact, even before the HCFA commenced such analyses there have been some studies likely aimed at classifying hospitals based on their mortality statistics. These studies linked death rates to some selected hospital characteristics, to patient volume and provider experience, but none of them sorted out inter-hospital death rate differentials according to the severity of illnesses involved, complexities of treatment especially invasive procedures, quality of care, or random selection factors[19]. Subsequently, it was shown that, at least partially, mortality rate differences could be attributed the differences in illness severity, such as in pneumonia, heart attacks, strokes, cancer, and the like often treated in intensive care units of the hospitals involved[20]. More recently, it was postulated that chance variations may account for a substantial portion of hospital death rate differences, also giving a significant role to differing levels of illness severities. Yet another study put most of the weight on illness severity related factors, lowering the significance of chance variations. One study suggested a connection between death rates and care quality based on peer review generated data on patients with pneumonia, stroke or heart attacks, suggesting twice as high a rate of preventable death occurrence in some hospitals than in others within the same hospital chain[21].

Although many of the hospital regulatory functions of the past, such as CON programs, have receded into the background and are in fact no longer used in many states, a brief look at how they related to mortality rates should constitute an interesting inquiry, and a basis for possible future policy decisions, should interest in these regulatory tools arise again. In addition, few studies have looked at the relationship between mortality rates and hospital ownership, and the relationship between mortality rates and the impact of competition. One study specifically looked at these issues for 16 selected conditions of some 215,000 patients from 981 hospitals covering most of the US from mid-1983 to mid-1984[22]. A significant direct or positive relationship was found between mortality rates and the stringency of state regulatory controls on price and by way of CON. The intensity of competition in the geographical regions was indicated by enrollment in HMOs, and that too showed a significant direct or positive relations with rates of mortality. No significant relationship was found between hospital ownership types and mortality rates, or between the latter and the number of hospitals competing in the immediate regional markets. These relationships suggest considerable support for strong quality assurance/control programs to accompany concentrated efforts aimed at containing costs or promoting competition.

Medicare Prospective Payment System and Hospital Care Quality

The implementation of the Medicare prospective payment system in 1983 [Public Law 98-21] may be seen as an incentive for hospitals to engage in at least two profit motivated endeavors: (a) cut costs to save money, perhaps on the expense of quality; (b) increase the volume of inpatient admissions, and the velocity of patient rotation (get them in, provide the minimum necessary care and get them out as soon as possible - increasing "patient velocity"). Under the traditional cost reimbursement system there was minimum or no incentive to control costs, for costs were reimbursed to the hospitals on a retrospective basis. Under a system where reimbursements are set prospectively, and the hospital knows in advance what it will get for each case [diagnosis], profit motive dictates that in view of the fixed revenue variable the various dimensions of the cost variables, including the patient's length of hospital stay, should be minimized. This process *could* take place at the expense of the patient and care quality could be compromised. Consequently, some organizations and researchers suggested that there was a need to take a closer look at the relationship between care quality and prospective payment system[23].

In spite of the interest in these issues, no formal methods or guidelines have been developed to pursue this matter. Thus, OTA indicates that "how hospitals and other providers actually will respond to the financial incentives inherent in PPS is by no means well understood ..."[24]. On the positive side, there may be a tendency on the part of hospitals to respond to PPS by specializing, each carving out its own area of expertise, increasing volume in that area of care endeavor, and hopefully increasing care quality due to increased experience and volume. While this would likely increase the quality of care in selected specialized and centralized institutions, it might compromise access to those services by patients located outside the hospital's region. Nonetheless, specialization would not likely reduce patient velocity, or patient velocity might remain unduly high. Subject to severity (case-mix) considerations and adjustments, the quality of PPS in this regard needs to be followed up by looking at post-hospital care facilities to which patients may readily, and at times prematurely, be discharged.

The inquiry into the quality consequences of PPS would need to cover at least three general areas: (a) access, (b) quality, (c) post-discharge environment. In relation to access, institutions would need to be identified who discriminate among patients based on the potential cost of treatment in favor of easier and less expensively treatable patients, and against more complex and potentially expensive treatment scenarios. Potentially high cost patients could either be not admitted or discharged prematurely. Average length of stay and admission rate trend differentials would give some indication of this predicament. Inpatient care quality might be compromised, as I suggested earlier, by simply cutting back on needed or unnecessary but nevertheless beneficial, such as ancillary, services to patients. Indicators of this predicament could include hospital specific mortality or early readmission rates, both of which have been discussed earlier. Finally, as to the post-discharge care environment, the concern is the time of discharge in comparison with what it would be under a retrospective reimbursement regime. At discharge a certain degree of patient dependency on hospital care may be identified. If that dependency is measurable and is noted at zero, then the discharge is not premature. The prematurity of the discharge may be thought to increase with this dependency factor. Once again, the extent to which PPS might have brought about premature discharge can be ascertained by comparing hospital specific dependency rates after PPS imposition with those prior to the PPS regime.

A relatively recent study examined the impact of PPS on hospital care quality, access and outcome by relying on an ongoing community-wide experiment in the City of Rochester NY during the 1980-84 time period[25]. It should be noted that at the beginning of this experiment Rochester was already below the national average in terms of hospital utilization and Medicare reimbursement costs, and these variables continued to improve during the duration of the experiment. Thus, between 1979 and 1983 hospitals that participated in the experiment experienced a 6% lower increase in costs than other hospitals in New York State, and 22% lower than hospitals in the rest of the country. During approximately the same period of time, Medicare reimbursements per beneficiary to these hospitals declined from 89% to 71% of the US average, ranking the City of Rochester in this regard much lower than most other cities in the US. Furthermore, admissions into these hospitals during the same period decreased from 134 to 124 and patient days by 3% per 1,000 population[26]. The study aimed to determine if the experimental prospective payment system during the early 1980s, notwithstanding, or perhaps because of, its favorable financial outcome had any negative impact on care quality or on access to care. The researchers, examining certain medical conditions only, found no significant evidence of a reduced care quality in connection with those conditions.

Whether the results of these experiments are readily applicable to Medicare's nation-wide cost containment efforts is questionable. The Rochester experiment with hospital reimbursements placed a maximum limit on total hospital expenditures and hospital-specific revenue minimums, discouraging unnecessary admissions and inpatient service utilization. The nation-wide Medicare reimbursement process, however, pays hospitals on a specific case-by-case diagnostic related group (DRG) basis, designed to limit inpatient hospital expenditures but may cause, as its revenue motivated by-product, increased admission frequencies. In addition, the Rochester experiment coordinated and oversaw all participating hospitals' activities through various organizations whose membership was made up of the participating hospitals themselves closely linking each others' operational and planning activities, not to be found in the national PPS regime.

Healthcare Quality at Nonhospital Institutional Providers

Healthcare cost containment policies of recent years, along with new diagnostic technology and increased competition in healthcare markets increased the presence of the so-called freestanding healthcare providers. These providers offer specialized healthcare services outside what we traditionally know as hospitals, physicians offices and nursing homes. Freestanding providers in most areas of the US normally include alcohol and drug abuse treatment centers, ambulatory care, psychiatric and surgical centers, chemo and radiation therapeutic cancer treatment centers, cardiac catheterization laboratories, comprehensive and specialized rehabilitation centers, diagnostic imaging centers, emergency centers, general diagnostic centers, home healthcare services, hospice care institutions, independent clinical laboratories, and pain control centers, among others.

The regulation of care quality provided by these clinics has for some time been of concern to healthcare policy analysts and policy makers. In particular, little is known about quality assurance programs that may be or could be implemented by these institutions. External quality assurance for providers such as these would include licensing, and the implementation and enforcement of regulatory efforts. It is far from being clear whether many of these freestanding providers have implemented internal quality assurance procedures, or that they even abide by external ones, or if they do, to what extent. It should nevertheless be noted that federal quality assurance standards have been established for some type of freestanding providers such as ambulatory surgi centers, home health agencies, clinical laboratories, comprehensive rehab centers, and hospices, if they seek to service Medicare patients. They are typically enforced by using state agencies for conducting inspections and determining compliance. Federal regulation does not reach freestanding providers if they do not serve Medicare patients, except that physicians are personally licensed. We will take a look at state initiated and implemented quality control measures later in this section. But first, we should note some internal quality control measures aimed at freestanding providers who service Medicare patients, for they do exist. These normally include a quality assurance plan, a complaint resolution system, peer review procedures and a continuous credentialing systems to ascertain up-to-date competence. Once again, while these measures are in place, the extent to which they are adhered to is uncertain, and for freestanding providers, their impact on quality has yet to be ascertained.

Let us now take a closer look at the role of states in overseeing care quality at freestanding providers[27]. In general, states impose quality assurance standards on freestanding providers if they also license them. Thus, quality of care scrutiny by the states of these providers is a function of licensing. Licensing requirements on the other hand are not uniform throughout the country, and in some states for certain types of services it is nonexistent. Where licensing does not exist, the state may simply not be aware of the provider's existence. Of the provider categories listed earlier, none were required to take out an operating license in Iowa and Vermont as of 1990, and at the other end of the scale, no more than nine were licensed in Massachusetts and Rhode Island. Alcohol and drug abuse centers operate in all of the states, and were required to be licensed in 42 as of 1987. The situation is similar for ambulatory surgical centers, and to a somewhat lesser extent for home health care organizations, hospice care and independent clinical laboratories. Chemotherapy and radiation cancer treatment, and pain control centers operated in about 16 states, all without licensing requirements. Of the 28 or so states where general diagnostic and diagnostic imaging centers operated, only three required licensing.

The writer is not aware of any significant up-to-date studies which take a further look at care quality and its enforcement in freestanding care providers. In fact, the issue seems to remain ominously aloof in comparison to care quality concerns at other providers discussed earlier.

Care Quality at Managed Care Organizations

Prepaid medical practice plans in the US have been in existence for many years. The Ross-Loos Clinic, and early versions of the plan, was founded in 1929. Other rather large plans which had been in existence for many years before HMOs became politically popular included Group Health of Puget Sound, Kaiser Permanente, Health Insurance Plan of Greater New York and the Harvard Community Health Plan. In 1973, Public-Law 93-222 was passed which provided funding for HMO development, and secured market access for HMOs by requiring employers to make HMOs as an option among health plans available to employees[28]. In return, the HMOs were to apply community-wide standards in rate setting and enrollment, and to provide a minimum set of basic but necessary services. HMO growth and development were accelerated by a 1976 Public-Law [94-460] which relaxed some of these constraints on HMOs. Legislative amendments relating to

HMOs in this time period allowed HMOs to benefit from secured markets and federal funding, government secured loans and managerial training, although some of these were discontinued later. Once much of the federal support was discontinued in the early 1980s, many HMOs became for-profit organizations and even publicly owned corporations.

Typically, and based upon functional and organizational factors, HMOs are grouped into four broad categories: staff, group, independent practice associations (IPAs) and network. In a *staff* model, physicians function as salaried employees, and the HMO as an organization assumes the financial risk for the care normally provided in HMO owned hospitals and clinics. In a *group* HMO, physicians organized in various types of group practice contract with the HMO to perform care services. An *IPA* is a separate legal entity that contracts with HMOs by offering otherwise separately and often individually practicing physicians' services, although lately it has not been unusual for IPAs to maintain their own HMOs. A *network* HMO delivers care by essentially franchising local HMOs, IPAs and other providers, and thus competes with other nonaffiliated providers in the regions involved.

Managed care and in particular various forms of HMOs have now become pervasive on the US healthcare scene. About 20% of the insured population was covered by HMO plans of one form or another. That represents a 100% increase during the preceding six years alone. IPAs, with over 60% of the enrollments, still appear to dominate the HMO scene, with the rest of the HMOs each having approximately the same share. Regionally, HMOs seem to concentrate in the mid-west with some 30% of the enrollees, relatively evenly distributed throughout the rest of the country. While initially most HMOs were non-profit institutions, recent years witnessed the emergence of for-profit organizations in a big way, with over 60% of HMOs becoming for-profit, although they have no more than about half of total membership. There has also been a significant increase in government's participation with HMOs. In recent years, there has been a close to 20% increase in Medicare beneficiary participation, and over 30% increase in Medicaid participants. In over half of the states, at least 10% of HMO enrollees constitute government sponsored health insurance beneficiaries, with Florida and California being the most predominant in this regard. The 2.2 million Medicare beneficiaries enrolled in various managed care environments constitute 6.3% of the total Medicare population. The largest jump in this regard took place between 1984 and 1987, when it almost doubled from 2.9% to 5.4%, contrasting with the increase to 6.3% between 1987 and

1992. In fact, in 1988 and 1989 the enrollment remained constant[29]. Nevertheless, this trend appears to continue, and as it does, governments will need to become increasingly concerned with the quality of care provided by HMOs.

The basic environment for classic HMO functioning may readily be seen as one conducive for healthcare quality deterioration. The capitated payment method provides an incentive for utilization control or even curtailment, allowing for absolutely necessary care only in situations where the margin for judgmental errors is minimal or non-existent. HMO affiliated physicians have often been and are given various financial incentives to control provider costs whether in the form of service or prescriptions. This has been viewed as a potential threat to care quality[30], although attempts have been made to mitigate the situation. Thus, when an HMO enters into a contract with Medicare, it needs to demonstrate a capability to comply with the Public Health Service Act and its standards in terms of management, internal quality assurance and financial solvency provisions. Until 1987, the HCFA, the government agency responsible for HMO provided healthcare quality for Medicare patients, attempted to monitor contracts with HMOs through its regional office network, and in particular through its Office of Prepaid Healthcare. Subsequently, and due to persistent problems as well as criticisms brought forth in another 1988 GAO Study[31] increased reliance was placed on contracted external Peer Review Organizations (PROs).

The PRO program was initially set up for Medicare contracted fee-for-service providers under TEFRA. PROs under contract with the Department of Health and Human Services reviewed the need, appropriateness and quality of inpatient services. HCFA's Bureau of Health Standards and Quality has been negotiating and monitoring PRO contracts. After January 1, 1987 all healthcare services rendered to Medicare patients were reviewed by PROs pursuant to the Consolidated Omnibus Budget Reconciliation Act of 1985 [Public Law 99-272, 1986]. Later in 1986, the Omnibus Budget Reconciliation Act of 1986 [Public-Law 99-509] amended the earlier 1986 COBRA provisions so that HCFA could contract with other reviewing entities, the so-called Quality Review Organizations (QROs) in addition to PROs to review HMO service quality. Other than the fact that QROs have not been called upon to review inpatient hospital services under the Medicare fee-for-service program, they were expected to perform the same functions as PROs in connection with HMOs, although to much more limited extent. However, by the time QRO contracting ceased altogether in late 1990 only one of them had a contract with HCFA, with the rest of the contracts having always been outstanding at PROs.

In early 1991, the USGAO issued a report on the performance of PROs by way of reviewing healthcare service quality rendered by HMOs to Medicare patients[32]. The Report concluded that HCFA has not adequately used PROs to ensure the presence of an effective Quality Assurance Program (QAP). One of the reasons for this inadequacy was that HCFA made it optional for HMOs to have their QAP reviewed by a PRO. Consequently, no more than 25% of the Medicare-participating HMOs had their QAPs reviewed by a PRO, and even of those that chose to be reviewed, half of the HMOs were "... unable to demonstrate the capability to identify and correct quality-of-care problems". Furthermore, it was noted at that time that "HCFA had no plans to have the PROs review all HMO internal QAPs or to evaluate the QAPs determined to be ineffective". The Report goes on further to note that "HCFA ... does not know how effective most HMO QAPs are at identifying and correcting quality problems. HCFA's own reviews of HMOs focus on the structural aspects of QAPs - that is, they attempt to validate the existence of a QAP rather than evaluate its effectiveness. HCFA could have required PROs to review the effectiveness of all QAPs as a way of complementing its own structural reviews, but made such evaluations optional. Most HMOs have chosen not to subject their QAP to PRO review"[33]. The situation presented appears to be even more serious when we are told by the report that "Neither the PROs nor the HCFA has acted to ensure that the HMOs correct the PRO-identified deficiencies in their QAPs. The PROs have no contractual requirement to follow up on these deficiencies to ensure that they are corrected, and PRO officials said they do not monitor HMO efforts to improve their QAPs because they lack the authority to enforce corrective action. None of the HMOs with a deficient QAP had requested the PRO to re-evaluate its program"[34].

The quality of HMO care performance, however, has not always been viewed negatively. Apart from professionals in the field who frequently give prepared statements at Congressional hearings[35], some healthcare research and policy scholars have also seen HMO performance in better or at least mixed lights. A study which covered a twenty year period from the late 1950s through the 1970s, assessing quality in terms of structure and process instead of outcome, found HMO care quality, at least in terms of their organization structure, impressive[36]. HMOs were now employing physicians who were younger with more up-to-date training. Yet, even then, several HMOs needed to rely on non-accredited hospitals and encountered difficulties in recruiting USD trained physicians[37]. Another major study which concentrated on one specific prepaid group practice, Group Health Cooperative of Puget Sound, a staff group practice type of HMO resemblance, found that patient costs were some 25% lower, while patient health outcomes were essentially the same as in fee-for-service environments[38]. Whether these positive assertions based on a study of one specific organization, which, incidentally, has even previously had a good reputation for cost savings and care quality, can be generalized to other prepaid group practices and HMOs is questionable.

Furthermore, the market environment in which HMOs have been forced to function has been drastically transformed since the mid-1980s when the Rand study was conducted. The HMO business is getting quite crowded. In the past HMOs were preoccupied with competing against fee-for-service plans with high fees and generally acceptable or accepted care quality. The competitive field has thus been relatively favorable for HMOs, at least from the point of view of the cost of care. Now, HMOs need to compete not only against fee-for-service providers but also quite emphatically among themselves as well as with other managed care providers in increasingly saturated markets. As managed care plans expand and attempt to compete, they will likely be less selective among those whom they enroll. Sicker patients will cost more money costing profits or compromising cost containment, with the latter less likely with also increasing corporate and otherwise coordinated healthcare purchasing powers. Thus, the HMO's relief valve may be sought in connection with the quality and the necessary quantity of the care rendered. It is possible that the largely untapped and probably increasing Medicare and Medicaid markets will cushion somewhat the competitive impact of the perpetual managed care expansion pressures, as indeed no more than 15% of Medicare and Medicaid beneficiaries are presently enrolled in HMOs. However, it is clearly a temporary solution, and given the GAO's findings regarding HMO quality enforcement measures under relatively relaxed HCFA and PRO monitoring, albeit some years ago, compounded by the fact that the cost of care for increasing numbers of elderly tends to be much higher than for younger patient populations, the question of care quality in connection with managed care organizations will likely be a topical concern for many years to come.

Notes

1. Arrow, K., "Uncertainty and the Welfare Economics of Medical Care", *American Economic Review,* Vol. 53, No. 5, 1963. See also Rosen, S., "Hedonic Prices and Implicit Markets: Product Differentiation in Pure Competition", *Journal of Political Economy,* Vol. 81, 1974.
2. Spence, A., "Job Market Signaling", *Quarterly Journal of Economics,* Vol. 87, No. 3, 1973, and "Premiums for High Quality Products as Returns to Reputation", *Quarterly Journal of Economics,* Vol. 98, No. 4, 1983. Akerlof, G., "Market for Lemons: Qualitative Uncertainty and the Market Mechanism", *Quarterly Journal of Economics,* Vol. 84, No. 3, 1970.
3. Hartz, A.J., Krakauer, H. et al., "Hospital Characteristics and Mortality Rates", *New England Journal of Medicine,* Vol. 321, 1989; DuBois, R.W., Brook, R.H., Rogers, W.H., "Adjusted Hospital Death Rates: A Potential Screen for Quality of Medical Care", *American Journal of Public Health,* Vol. 77, 1987. See also Feingenson, J.S., Feigenson, W.D., et al., "Outcome and Cost for Stroke Patients in Academic and Community Hospitals: A Comparison of Two Groups Referred to Regional Rehabilitation Center", *JAMA,* Vol. 240, 1978; Morehead, M.A., *A Study of Hospital Care Secured by a Sample of Teamster Family Members in New York City,* Columbia School of Public Health and Administrative Medicine, New York, 1964; Safran, C., Phillips, R.S., "Intervention to Prevent Readmission: The Constraints of Cost and Efficacy", *Medical Care,* Vol. 27, 1989; Bigby, J., Dunn, J. et al., "Assessing the Preventability of Hospital Emergency Admission", *American Journal of Medicine,* Vol. 83, 1986; Mason, W.B., Bedwell, C.L., Vander-Zwaag, R., Runyan, J.W., "Why People are Hospitalized: A Description of Preventable Factors Leading to Admission for Medical Illness", *Medical Care,* Vol. 18, 1980; and Jencks, S.F., Williams, D.K., Kay, T.L., "Assessing Hospital Associated Death from Discharge Data: The Role of Length of Stay and Comorbidities", *JAMA,* Vol. 260, 1988.
4. Park, R.E., Brook, R.H. et al., "Explaining Variations in Hospital Death Rates: Randomness, Severity of Illness, and Quality of Care", *JAMA,* Vol. 264, 1990. Green, J., Wintfeld, N., Sharkey, P., Passman, L.J., "The Importance of Severity of Illness in Assessing Hospital Mortality", *JAMA,* Vol. 263, 1990. Berwick, D.M., Wald, D.L., "Hospital Leaders' Opinions of the HFCA's Mortality Data", *JAMA,* Vol. 263, 1990.
5. Kahn, K.L., Rubenstein, L. V. et al., "The Effects of the DRG-based Prospective Payment System on Quality of Care for Hospitalized Patients: An Introduction to the Series", *JAMA,* Vol. 264, 1990. Brennan, T.A., Localio, A.R., Laird, N.M., "Reliability and Validity of Judgments Concerning Adverse Events and Negligent Care Suffered by Hospitalized Patients", *Medical Care,* Vol. 29, 1989.
6. Brennan, T.A., Herbert, L.E. et al., "Hospital Characteristics Associated With Adverse Events and Substandard Care", *JAMA,* Vol. 265, 1991.
7. DesHarnais, S.I., McMahon, L.F. et al., "The Development and Variation of Risk-Adjusted Indexes of Mortality, Readmissions, and Complications", *Medical Care,* Vol. 28, 1990.
8. DesHarnais, S. et al., "The Risk-adjusted Mortality Index: A New Measure of Hospital Performance", *Medical Care,* Vol. 25, 1988.
9. Iezzone, L.I., Restuccia, J.D. et al., "The Utility of Severity of Illness Information in Assessing the Quality of Hospital Care", *Medical Care,* Vol. 30, 1992.
10. Thomas, J.W., Holloway, J.J., "Investigating Early Readmission as an Indicator for Quality of Care Studies", *Medical Care,* Vol. 29, 1991.

11. Sloan, F.A., Feidman, R.D. and Steinwald, A.B., "Effects of Teaching on Hospital Care", *Journal of Health Economics*, Vol. 2, 1983. Richard, T., Lurie, N. et al., "Measuring Differences Between Teaching and Nonteaching Hospitals", *Medical Care*, Vol. 26 (Supp), 1988. Garber, A.M., Fuchs, V.R., Silverman, J.F., "Case-mix, Cost and Outcome", *New England Journal of Medicine*, Vol. 310, 1984; and Relman, A.S., "Who Will Pay for Medical Education in Our Teaching Hospitals", *Science*, Vol. 226, 1984.

12. Boice, J.L., McGregor, M., "Effect of Residents' Use of Laboratory Tests on Hospital Costs", *Journal of Medical Education*, Vol. 58, 1983; Hueston, W.J., "Influence of a Family Practice Residency on Costs of Inpatient Diagnostic Testing", *Journal of Family Practice*, Vol. 23, 1986.

13. Shortell, S.M., Hughes, E.F.X., "Effects of Regulation, Competition, and Ownership on Mortality Rates Among Hospital Inpatients", *New England Journal of Medicine*, Vol. 318, 1988; Wennberg, J.E., Roos, N. et al., "Use of Claims Data Systems to Evaluate Healthcare Outcomes", *JAMA*, Vol. 257, 1987; Fletcher, R.H., O'Malley, M.S., Ear, J.A., "Patients' Priorities for Medical Care", *Medical Care*, Vol. 21, 1983.

14. Rich, E.C., Gifford, G. et al., "The Relationship of House Staff Experience to the Cost and Quality of Inpatient Care", *JAMA*, Vol. 263, 1990.

15. Hartz, A.J., Krakauer, H. et al., "Hospital Characteristics and Mortality Rates", *New England Journal of Medicine*, Vol. 321, 1989; and Kuhn, E.M., Hartz, A.J. et al., "Relationship of Hospital Characteristics and the Results of Peer Review in Six Large States", *Medical Care*, Vol. 29, 1990.

16. US Congress, *Medicare's Disproportionate Share Adjustment for Hospitals*, US Congressional Budget Office, Washington, DC, 1990. Epstein, A.M., Stern, R.S., Weissman, J.S., "Do the Poor Cost More? A Multihospital Study of Patients' Socioeconomic Status and Use of Hospital Resources", *New England Journal of Medicine*, Vol. 322, 1990. Thorpe, K.E., "Why Are Urban Hospital Costs So High? The Relative Importance of Patient Source of Admission, Teaching Competition, and Case Mix", *Health Services Research*, Vol. 22, 1988. Also see Medicaid Catastrophic Act of 1988, 1395ww USC 42.

17. Burstin, H.R., Lipsitz, S.R. et al., "Socioeconomic Status and Risk for Substandard Medical Care", *JAMA*, Vol. 268, 1992.

18. Burstin, H.R., Lipsitz, S.R. et al., "The Effect of Hospital Financial Characteristics on Quality of Care", *JAMA*, Vol. 270, 1993.

19. Fink, A., Yano, E.M., Brook, R.H., The Condition of the Literature on Differences in Hospital Mortality", *Medical Care*, Vol. 27, 1989. Riley, G., Lubitz, J., "Outcomes of Surgery Among the Medicare Aged: Surgical Volume and Mortality", *Health Care Financing Review*, Vol. 7, 1985. Luft, H.S., Bunker, J.P., Enthoven, A.C., "Should Operations Be Regionalized? The Empirical Relation Between Surgical Volume and Mortality", *New England Journal of Medicine*, Vol. 301, 1979. Flood, A.B., Scott, W.R., Ewy, W., "Does Practice Make Perfect? [*Part I*: The Relation Between Hospital Volume and Outcomes for Selected Diagnostic Categories. *Part II*: The Relation Between Volume and Outcomes and Other Hospital Characteristics]", *Medical Care*, Vol. 22, 1984.

20. Greenfield, S., Aronow, H.U. et al., "Flaws in Mortality Data: the Hazards of Ignoring Comorbid Disease", *JAMA*, Vol. 260, 1988. DuBois, R.W., Rogers, W.H. et al., "Hospital Inpatient Mortality: Is it a Predictor of Quality?", *New England Journal of Medicine*, Vol. 317, 1987.

21. Jencks, S.F., Daley, J. et al., "Interpreting Hospital Mortality Data: The Role of Clinical Risk Adjustment", *JAMA*, Vol. 260, 1988. Green, J., Wintfeld, N. et al.,

"The Importance of the Severity of Illness in Assessing Hospital Mortality", *JAMA*, Vol. 263, 1990. Also see DuBois in N. 20.

22.   See Seplaki, L., *Cost and Competition in American Medicine: Theory, Policy and Institutions*, University Press of America, Lanham, MD, 1994, Ch 12.

23.   Lohr, K.N., Brook, R.H. et al., *Impact of Medicare Prospective Payment System on the Quality of Medical Care: A Research Agenda*, The Rand Corporation, Publication No. R-3242-HCFA, March 1995. See also, *Prospective Payment Assessment Commission*, Report and Recommendation to the Secretary, US Department of Health and Human Services, April 1986. Office of Technology Assessment, US Congress. *Medicare Prospective Payment System: Strategies for Evaluating Cost, Quality and Medical Technology*, Publication No. OTA-H-263, US Government Printing Office, Washington, DC, 1985. And, General Accounting Office, *Efforts to Evaluate Medicare Prospective Payment Effects are Insufficient*, Pub. No. GAO/PEMD-86-10, US Government Printing Office, Washington, DC, 1986. See also, *Medicare Quality of Care and Outcomes and Effectiveness Research*, Hearing Before the Subcommittee on Health of the Committee on Ways and Means, House of Representatives, 102nd Congr, First Session, April 30, 1991.

24.   See OTA cited in 23.

25.   Mushlin, A.I., Panzer, R.J. et al., "Quality of Care During a Community-Wide Experiment in Prospective Payment to Hospitals", *Medical Care*, Vol. 26, 1988.

26.   Block, J.A., Regenstreif, D.I., Griner, P.F., "A Community Hospital Payment Experiment Outperforms National Experience: The Hospital Experimental Payment Program in Rochester, NY", *JAMA*, Vol. 257, 1987. American Hospital Association, *Hospital Statistics, Years 1980-85*, AHA, Chicago, IL. McClure, W., Shaller, D., "Datawatch: Variations in Medicare Expenditures", *Health Affairs*, Vol. 3, 1984. All cited in 24.

27.   Much of this section is based on a GAO study of 1990. United States General Accounting Office, Report to the Chairman, Subcommittee on Health and Longterm Care, Select Committee on Aging, House of Representatives. *Health Care: Limited State Efforts to Assure Quality of Care Outside Hospitals*, GAO/HRD-90-53, January 1990.

28.   Seplaki, L., *Cost and Competition in American Medicine: Theory, Policy and Institutions*, University Press of America, Lanham, MD, 1994, Ch 14.

29.   See note 27. See also, "Growth in Medicare Health Maintenance Organization Enrollment: CY 1992", *Health Care Financing Review, Medicare and Medicaid Statistical Supplement*, HCFA Publication No. 03348, February 1995.

30.   United States General Accounting Office [GAO], *Medicare: Physician Incentive Payments by Prepaid Health Plans Could Lower Quality of Care*, GAO/HRD-89-29, December 12, 1988.

31.   *GAO. Medicare: Experience Shows Ways to Improve Oversight of Health Maintenance Organizations*, GAO/HRD-88-73, August 1988.

32.   United States General Accounting Office, Report to the Ranking Minority Member, Special Committee on Aging, United States Senate, *Medicare: PRO Review Does Not Assure Quality of Care Provided by Risk HMOs*, GAO/HRD-91-48, March 1991.

33.   See note 32, Ch 2, p. 17-18.

34.   See note 32, p. 22.

35.   See for instance, *Medicare HMO's and Quality Assurance: Unfulfilled Promises*, Hearing before the Special Committee on Aging, United States Senate, 102nd Congress, 1st Session, March 1991, Washington, DC, where several professionals

from the industry presented prepared statements by way of attempts to clarify or outright contradict the GAO's position.

36. Cunningham, F. and Williamson, J., "How Does the Quality of Care in HMOs Compare to that in Other Settings? An Analytic Literature Review: 1958-1979", *Group Health Journal,* Vol. 1, Winter 1980.

37. Luft, H.S., "HMOs and the Quality of Care", *Inquiry,* Vol. 25, Spring 1988.

38. Ware, J.E. et. al., "Comparison of Health Outcomes at a Health Maintenance Organization With Those of Fee-for-Service", *Lancet,* May 1986. See also statement "It is unclear whether the cost reductions in HMOs, which are achieved largely by reductions in hospital admissions, have adverse effects on health" in Ware, J.E., Rodgers, W.H. et al., R-3459-HHS, The Rand Corporation, Santa Monica CA, October 1987.

7 Healthcare Quality and The Individual Provider

In general, it is reasonable to assume that physician performance in terms of both quantity and quality is heavily influenced by the potential income of the provider, the amount and the timing of the payments involved, indirect financial incentives that may be present, and by the institutional environment in which the care service is supplied, i.e. in private solo practice, fee-for-service group, or managed care type of prepaid group. Some proof of how physicians actually perform under these circumstances and for the various business and professional motives could be generated by relevant empirical studies, much of which appears to be absent from the literature. Even what is there dates back to pre-1983 periods when the medical scene was different from the way it has evolved in recent years. All of the general factor categories enumerated above have been changing. The Medicare Prospective Payment System altered the mode of payment for hospital inpatient care, and presumably the motive for and delivery of care as well. The Resource Based Relative Value Scale (RBRVS) physician payment system under Medicare's Part B also transformed relevant physician price structures prompting a potential redistribution of providers among the various traditional and new speciality groups. Pervasive managed care environments slowly engulfing individual practitioners contain various financial incentives which could have direct and indirect effect on both the quantity and, particularly by way of timing, the quality of care delivered. Solo practice appears at least at the present to be on the way out. Group practice on the other hand appears to be on the increase.

Since financial variables are paramount determinants of most physicians' practice dimensions, they will impact on the *quality* and *quantity* of service which physicians will perform with the understanding that at least these two dimensions are by no means independent. Thus, if physicians receive a fixed fee for each unit of service rather than a fixed amount for each episode of illness or patient, the volume and frequency of service units will likely rise by the maximum number of units which the physician perceives as consistent with standards of care and subject to ethical constraints. Changing physician payment schemes may prompt a change in the quality of care by way of altered service requests on behalf of the patient, by physicians not accepting assignment forcing the patient to seek out less expensive potentially less adequate care provided by less qualified personnel, by forcing practitioners out of solo practice into group affiliated managed care environments, and constraining providers in terms of their location and specialization choices as well in terms of their diligence to keep up with the state of the art in diagnostic and therapeutic care categories as well as in terms of the technologies involved.

The Physician: Whose Agent?

The structure of medical care delivery presumes that in most cases the care administered to the patient including the process, location and manner whereby that care is administered is at least initially determined or strongly suggested by the physician. The reason being that the patient simply does not have the knowledge and information so as to arrive at a proper diagnosis, determination of care need, available care alternatives, potential outcomes and other important information variables which, if present, would enable the patient to arrive at some informed decisions as to care choice and various cost/price alternatives in view of discernible quality. In other words, the patient is typically at the complete disposal of the provider's decision in terms of care administration which places the provider in a double-agent position: that for the patient and for the provider's self. The provider is to make patient-specific care decisions subject to his/her profession's ethical constraints which in principle normally place the patient's interest in a position of paramount importance, far above those of the provider's own personal or financial interests. Thus, a physician is called upon to be a "perfect agent" of the patient to be governed only by the patient's interest and not at all by that of the physician, constrained in the delivery of care only by community-wide accepted medical standards and his or her own competence. However, negative externalities may impact upon the practice of medicine. We have already pointed to possible cost constraint efforts, and institutionally imposed financial incentives to curtail care. The threat of medical malpractice on the other hand may conflict with these considerations, causing the provider to produce more rather than less care by way of practicing so called "defensive medicine"[1].

In addition to decisions made by the provider, patient decisions may also impact upon the quality of care. Patients themselves have financial incentives and constraints. They have personal dispositions to healthcare acquired through their social and economic environments, and strongly influenced by cultural and in some cases religious considerations. Thus, if a patient has to pay more for care due to increases in coinsurance less care may be sought[2]. Increases in provider fees or non-acceptance of Medicare assignments will also channel patients to alternative groups of providers, or to none at all. Over time, however, all of these factors influencing patient outlook regarding care are liable to change, hence their impact upon the demand for healthcare should be examined in a dynamic context.

Thus far we referred to physician-specific issues, namely, those that arise from within the practice environment of the individual provider, and are driven by the direct financial, personal and professional interests of the provider. There are exogenous factors which also impact upon physician practice. Thus, the medical market itself may impact on physician practice patterns and *modus operandi*. Within specific community settings, physicians may employ various methods to compete for patients. These methods have been found to include price competition, quality image creating campaigns, advertising through office windows and the media, and outright adverse personal contacts and various forms of direct and indirect pressure. Intra-community inter-provider litigation motivated largely by competitive or economic factors is not uncommon. A fee-for-service based physician will competitively consider the practice patterns and fee structure of other similar practitioners, and will likely experience fee pressures from neighboring managed care-based practices as well. It may be that under these circumstances practice patterns tend towards a uniformity within each community since service inferiorities or financial adversities of one practice will cause a migration of patients to another practice in the same community and the losing practices may consider adopting the *modus operandi* of those that gain. This assumes perfect information in community-based medical markets on the part of both the patients and the practices, the former to determine the direction of migration, the latter to make the necessary adjustment in practice patterns.

The function of a physician as a "perfect agent" for the patient also includes full consideration of the patient's financial status, as well as the health status indicated earlier. In general, the market price of an input into any production process reflects its value to society, its opportunity cost. The presence of insurance coverage and various tax policies cause a divergence between the social cost and the price of medical care to the patient. The price of the care to the patient is lower than its social cost, and this divergence may also impact upon physicians' care service input decisions. Hence, if the physician were to follow economic convention and input care up to the point where the marginal benefit of the care to the patient is equal to its marginal cost (price) to the patient, then probably under-treatment would result, and the quality of care even in terms of structure and process would likely be negatively impacted. The remedy for insurance covered services would then appear to be an over-supply of those care services commensurate with community standards of medical practice[3]. Thus, while the physician may succeed at functioning as the patient's "perfect" agent, it may not be viewed as such from society's point of view. The practice environment may also be an important factor in this respect.

Organizational and Financial Determinants of Physician Provided Care

It is possible that care provided by physicians in large group practice differs in a number of ways from that provided by a solo practitioner. The source of this difference, however, may be difficult to identify for it could be due to the manner whereby physicians are paid, or to their respective practice organization, the type of utilization controls applied, financial incentives available to the patients as well as to physicians in addition to their basic remuneration structure, and so forth. Furthermore, there may be significant quality differences among practitioners even within the various practice categories, i.e. care quality among solo practitioners may likely differ, and so would quality among members of any group practice. In general, it is likely that physician remuneration practices will affect the quality of care given through provider choice of services offered, the decision whether or not to hospitalize, to utilize specialized services, whether or not to recommend surgery, and the utilization of some possibly essential diagnostic test alternatives. In this context the quality of patient care is reduced when either irrelevant or inconsequential services, particularly with considerable risk to the patient, are provided, or when services that would be beneficial to the patient are not provided[4].

In a *traditional* **fee-for-service** environment, Medicare paid the provider for services rendered in various care-specific coded categories, based on what has been considered as "customary, prevailing and reasonable" and adjusted periodically as well as regionally by region-specific economic indexes. In this manner local price structures evolved that were case, region and speciality-specific, constrained by economic indexes. This structure in turn prompted practice and utilization patterns which yielded the highest financial return to the provider, caused speciality shifts into higher paying fields of endeavors, and regional shifts into financially and socio-economically more favored areas of the country away from less favorable ones, leaving some regions of the country without adequate care both in terms of quality and quantity. Thus, physicians received higher per time and effort unit fees for more technical procedures such as surgery and various forms of endoscopies than for simple patient consultations and preliminary diagnostic examinations. This prompted a shift into these higher paid more sophisticated areas and reduced emphases on and interest in lower paid practice. In fact, an entire image and prestige shift appears to have occurred in favor of these higher paid specialities[5].

In addition the these problems, fees implemented for new complex procedures remained relatively high in comparison with older procedures even though expertise and efficiency may have increased, hence time, effort and related costs decreased with experience. Furthermore, urban fee structures were generally higher than rural ones causing an influx of qualified physicians into metropolitan areas, leaving rural populations without adequate qualified care. As part of a related set of problems, metropolitan areas usually with university affiliated medical centers, provided much more by way of possibilities and facilities for specialization, which, given the higher fees for various sophisticated specialities tended to shift many practitioners away from the general practice of medicine into these areas of specialization. Thus, we had developed an urban concentration of specialists and a rural scarcity for even adequate care.

The fee structures themselves had various inherent problems which tended to elevate care costs, without necessarily improving quality. Given service unit-specific rates, physician income could be increased by simply producing more units of a given service, either by requesting patient return visits or producing service units to newly recruited patients[6]. Service units could also be coded or recoded so as to fall into a higher rate category, without any positive impact on the patient's health status. In addition, so called "unbundling" of services could be implemented whereby the total income received for the sum of the separated service components is greater than if the service bundle was to be covered by a single fee; thus, a diagnostic x-ray procedure may have in the past been included in the total service fee, but once separated out it would be charged for separately without reducing the original charge for the office visit.

While the result of this predicament is likely to be higher physician revenue hence higher costs, their impact on care quality and access is less certain, and depends on a number of factors. Thus, patients with complete insurance coverage and no deductibles or co-payments may not directly be affected by the various income inducing practices available to physicians. Patients, however, with co-payments and significant deductibles will directly feel the increase in the cost of their care and may decide to delay seeking care or stay away altogether, unless compelling situations arise. This impacts upon access and could ultimately reduce the quality of care, particularly as measured by outcome when the latter is influenced by the timing of care commencement in the first place, such as in severe cases of infection, pneumonia, or cancer.

The result of fee-for-service or extensive Medicare reimbursement systems could be an *over or under supply* of provider services. Oversupply of service occurs when the patient is subjected to care items which are redundant and are at best neutral for the patient's health status. Undersupply occurs when services with substantial benefits are not provided. Studies which attempt to determine the extent of oversupply would examine treated populations and the need for the services rendered. Thus, these studies may be relatively easy to undertake since the populations is defined as those having been subjected to the treatment or care items. Undersupply of care is a more difficult area to study for here the population may need to include people who were not treated but should have been, people who have not received certain care items but should have, people for whom there is no record of treatment when there should be one. That is, the population is more difficult to identify or delineate empirically, and there is no specific sample of people such as those found in connection with discerning oversupply of care. In addition, some areas of medical care supply are more likely to be scrutinized than others, depending upon the extent to which patients make use of available care. Care items covered by insurance, or services rendered to inpatients which are technical and complex in nature, such as surgical procedures, care items which patients use without direct financial constraints, all tend to be more available for scrutiny than services rendered in other circumstances. Indeed, most empirical studies published on care quality in a fee-for-service setting tend to use surgical and other care rendered in inpatient settings.

A number of studies have attempted to ascertain whether or not service quality differences may exist among areas of physician *specialization*, and whether care quality improves with specialization. The notion of specialization itself is several decades old. Many years ago, the typical physician would graduate from medical school and would commence "general practice" after a year of internship or some form of other hands-on training, while only a relatively few would pursue several years of additional training in order to become specialized. During the past two decades, this trend changed with more physicians specializing in some area or another, in fact, many developed and trained for sub-specialities within their specific speciality (e.g. some orthopedists work on shoulders only while others concentrate on knees) and less remaining in the traditional general practice of medicine. Earlier studies suggested a general positive relationship between the number of years in post-medical school training and the quality of service rendered. More recent studies looked at specifics in various inpatient and ambulatory settings and found a positive relationship between the training necessitated by board certification and the quality of care - when compared to the performance of similar care items by non-certified practitioners, although the certification itself in contrast to the prerequisite training did not appear to be a decisive factor. In addition, care generated within specialities was found to be better than when the same physicians functioned outside their specialities[7].

Physician Performance Under the Medicare Fee Schedule - the Early Years

For about a quarter of a century, physicians were reimbursed by Medicare based on "customary, prevailing, and reasonable" (CPR) fee criteria, which reflected local regionally based fee trends. In 1989, an important part of The Omnibus Budget Reconciliation Act [OBRA - Public Law 101-293] fundamentally changed this payment system which tended to overpay technical procedures such as surgery, anesthesiology and other procedures of a more complex nature and underpay more cognitive and intuitive services such as office visits and others normally found in general/family practice. With the *magnitude* of relative work effort set as the basis for reimbursement, fees in general were altered in favor of office visits and against surgeries as well as a number of diagnostic tests. In particular, fees are set by a resource-based relative value scale (RBRVS) first developed at Harvard and then revised and refined by the Physician Payment Review Commission (PPRC) and HCFA. HCFA suggested that the new system would significantly alter income distribution among various groups of practicing physicians, with as yet uncertain conclusions regarding care quality and outcome[8]. Historically this legislation implemented the most fundamental set of changes in physician payment policy since 1965, when Medicare itself was enacted. To be sure, there were other efforts in the past to control physician reimbursements by Medicare. The Medicare Economic Index was initiated in 1975 which was also aimed at limiting increases in physician reimbursements. On several occasions, various incentive programs were offered to physicians to induce assignment acceptance. The 1987, "maximum allowable actual charge limits" constrained nonparticipating physician charges to Medicare patients. In 1989 and 1990, fee schedules were initiated for radiology and anesthesiology, respectively. However, none of these had or will likely have the impact upon the physician reimbursement system which the current reform is likely to have.

The 1989 OBRA medical payment reform has several major phases, including the Medicare fee schedule (MFS), constraining physician billing beyond the official fee schedule, setting growth rate targets for physician fee payments, or volume performance standards. A 10% bonus is paid to physicians practicing in otherwise healthcare shortage areas. No fee differences will prevail among specialities in specific geographical areas. The reforms were in large part motivated by the rapidly increasing physician component of total healthcare expenditures. In fact, while total healthcare expenditures in general have about tripled during the past decade, the physician component of those expenditures have almost quadrupled during the same time. The alternatives for controlling the physician expenditure component included capitated payments, negotiated fees, and the recently developed payment reforms. According to a 1992 Report of the Physician Payment Review Commission (PPRC), expenditures for physician services within the Medicare program have increased at an average annual rate of some 13% since 1965. Thus, physician reimbursements constituted some 70% of Medicare's Part B, and over 25% of total Medicare expenditures. In addition, Medicare's traditional reimbursement system based on the so called customary, prevailing and reasonable (CPR) reimbursement system generated gross inequities among fees and income levels among various specialities, procedure types and different geographical regions. These inequities were not justified by the various inputs needed to perform those services. The payment reform is designed to make physician reimbursements based on service, specialities, and locations more equitable. It utilizes estimated *resource costs* that go into the service, instead of *charges* that constituted the basis for reimbursement under the traditional CPR system; the latter provided the incentive to increase the supply of costly surgical and diagnostic procedures on the expense of primary care items. Furthermore, according to PPRC's 1992 Report, so called "balanced billing", i.e. physician charges to Medicare beneficiaries beyond Medicare's maximum reimbursement levels has reached almost 20% of household income, doubling over the past decade. Thus, through the 1989 OBRA and as part of the overall medical fee schedule (MFS), which includes various payment system provisions and physician payment policies, physician service fees were derived utilizing a resource-based relative value system (RBRVS), cost control mechanisms were implemented by way of so called Medicare volume performance standards (MVPS), and ceilings were placed on balance billing by non-participating providers. RBRVS is a methodological foundation for the MFS, and takes into consideration total physician work, practice expenses, and malpractice coverage costs. The components are measured in relative value units (RVUs) which represent the physician's input in terms of time, skill and physical as well as mental efforts, stress and various uncontrollable risks. Physician fee setting utilize these RVUs derived from the RBRVS after geographical cost difference adjustments, and the actual dollar amounts are a product of the application of national conversion factors. Physicians' actual reimbursable service fees are calculated by using the following equation: $FEE_{i;L} = [CF]$ $[(GAF_{i;L}) (RVU_{w, I} + RVU_{pe, I} + RVU_{m, i})]$ where i is the ith service item, GAF is an adjustment factor for specific procedures or locations and is made up of the weighted average of the physician effort, practice expense, and malpractice expense components (expressed in terms of Geographic Practice Cost Indexes, or GPCIs); CF is the national conversion factor used to convert the three indicated relative value units (RVUs), weighted by their respective GAF indexes, into monetary terms. The sum of the three RVUs comprise Medicare's total RVU. The three RVUs in the formula are resource component specific that went into the RBRVS calculations for a service item i, i.e. w - specific work involved, pe - practice expense, and m - medical malpractice coverage. Thus, each RVU varies by procedure, and for each specific procedure there is a location-specific GAF, where L designates one of the 200 Medicare pricing locations.

Much of the Medicare fee schedule was implemented on January 1, 1992, although the transition of complete implementation will continue through 1996. The new payment system will ultimately redistribute some income to primary care services and into rural regions. Earlier noted HFCA simulations predicted an overall +10% to −15% range for a change in physician reimbursements by Medicare for the first year, 1992, embedding within this range substantial variations by practice speciality and geography. The

MFS includes a Geographic Practice Cost Index (GPCI) designed to adjust for geographical practice cost differences, and by allowing only for 25% of these differences Congress further sought to reduce the payment disparities between urban (the traditionally higher payment areas) and rural population regions.

As part of the 1989 OBRA, Congress requires the HHS to monitor and report annually to Congress on the impact of the new Medicare physician payment system. In particular, changes in healthcare service utilization and access to healthcare services are monitored pursuant to the new system. However, even before adequate data is gathered for more concrete empirical observations and studies, some likely consequences may be projected. There are likely to be shifts in both the demand for and the supply of physician services in the various areas of medical endeavor. The supply of some services will most likely be affected by the reduction or elimination of price differentials as well as by the billing constraints on physicians. "Compensating supply manipulations" may occur by an increase in the supply of services for which fees have been reduced, limit care for Medicare patients with more resources allocated to paying patients, or change the service-bundle for Medicare patients such as charging separately for initial consultations and increase the number of preprocedure consultations in surgical cases, which in the past would have normally been included in the overall fee. Consumer demand may be altered if out-of-pocket costs change. Changes in coinsurance will likely generate corresponding changes in the quantity of care service units demanded, and an increased use of so called "medigap" policies designed to take up excesses beyond Medicare reimbursements to physicians might also stimulate demand for care.

Since the early stages of the physician payment reform implementation, HCFA submitted four Annual Reports to Congress on monitoring the reform's impact on utilization and access, with the fifth Report expected out during the latter part of 1995. The first two reports dealt with preliminary matters such as designs and analytical approaches to the monitoring process, and data sources, with the second Report also having examined patterns physician service use under Medicare B during the period preceding the payment reform's implementation, since no experience data was yet available for the implementation of the new system itself. The 1993 Report does contain some preliminary data yielded by the monitoring system for 1992, the first full year of implementation. The 1994 Report contains eight separate studies to develop information about access to care in the periods before and after the introduction of the Medicare fee schedule, and will be dealt with in greater detail in the next section of this chapter[9].

The *1993 Report* reflects on a monitoring process of the payment reform's impact upon the system largely in terms of two broad dimensions: access and utilization, relying on baseline comparisons, i.e. comparative trends prior to and subsequently the reform's implementation, and six analyses. In addition to comparative trend analyses, the impact of the payment reform is also being monitored in relation to special patient groups such as minorities, rural, low-income, and the elderly who may have been disadvantaged in terms of some aspects of access and utilizations even before the new MFSs were implemented in 1992. The actual monitoring process relies on data from HCFA's Medicare *National Claims History* database (NCH) which since 1990 was modified to receive claims data daily from HCFA's nine so called "host sites" which approve claims submitted to them by the previously existing fiscal agents who, in turn, receive the claims directly from the providers themselves. This process keeps the datafile current, and the NCH is the primary source of Medicare Part B utilization data, based on the beneficiary as the unit of analysis, and containing data for various Medicare population groups and subgroups classified by various dimensions of geography, age, nature of the claim, and a host of other parameters included in the claims form. The beneficiary based files in the NCH are supplemented by two provider-based datafiles, also relying on all of the data submitted to NCH on the Medicare claims. The physician-supplier procedure summary file monitors physician category-specific service and payment changes by speciality and geography. The other file contains physician-specific data on payments and service patterns for a sample representing about 5% of the physician population.

All physicians caring for Medicare beneficiaries are registered and uniquely identified in the Medicare Physician Identification and Eligibility System, which assigns physicians a unique physician identifier number (UPIN), also entered by providers on the claims for reimbursement. Care services provided by physicians are classified into a HCFA Common Procedure Coding System (HCPCS) containing some 7, 000 codes for all procedures and services normally delivered, although the coding system is a dynamic one in that it is continuously undergoing various revisions and adjustments. The six analyses on the various aspects of access and utilization monitoring in the 1993 report mentioned earlier either present preliminary data from the monitoring process for the year 1992, or analyze baseline trends for periods prior to the 1992 implementation. The results for 1992, the first full year of implementation, were clearly preliminary although played some role in assessing the early impact of the payment reform on access and utilization in relation to baseline years.

Care Service and the Payment Reforms: HCFA's 1994 Report to Congress

During late 1994, HCFA submitted its fourth and most recent report to Congress regarding the results of its monitoring the physician payment reform impact upon care, access and various dimensions of utilization. The report, based on eight separate studies, is divided into three sections; a discussion of changes and related issues in the payment system, findings, and conclusions. The 1994 report confirms the findings of the previous year's report to the effect that the new payment policies did bring about the intended changes, although differences among some socio-economic groups in terms access to care do seem to persist.

As indicated earlier the 1989 Omnibus Budget Reconciliation Act (OBRA) of 1989 [Public Law 101-239] enacted the most important set of changes in Medicare B since the program started back in 1966. Section 1848(g)(7) of the Social Security Act mandates the Secretary of DHHS to monitor and report annually to Congress changes in care utilization and access in terms of various dimensions, such as population groups geographical areas, and types of service. The medical fee schedule (MFS) was largely implemented in 1992, with the implementation process scheduled to be completed by 1996. Limits were placed on physician charges beyond the MFS, and target rates of growth were imposed on total physician reimbursements. All for the purpose of reducing the difference in physician fees and income between those providing primary care and various specialists, and among various geographical areas. In the latter dimension, fees are allowed to differ only to the extent of reflecting differing practice costs. The new system lowered the fees of specialists [particularly those in surgery] in urban areas and positively adjusted those for primary care providers in rural regions of the country. In general, the relative fee and earnings tend towards equality among specialities and geographical areas. A bonus of 10% of set levels was implemented to encourage practice in so called health professional shortage areas. I also noted that the 1989 OBRA was not the first attempt at reforming physician payment systems so as to affect access and utilization. In 1975, the Medicare Economic Index set a limit on fee increases. In 1984, a physician Medicare participation inducement program was implemented to encourage physicians to participate in the program. In 1987, the Maximum Allowable Actual Charge (MAAC) provision limited nonparticipating physician fees charged to Medicare beneficiaries. In 1988 and 1990, downward adjustments were implemented in reimbursements for some procedures that were considered too expensive at the time. Finally, official fee schedules were implemented for radiology and anesthesiology in 1989 and 1990, respectively. Thus, as in connection with general healthcare reform efforts and attempts in the past which attempts are likely to be perennially repeated in the future, reforms of physician payment systems should also be viewed as a continuing dynamic process which will unlikely arrive at a permanently optimum solution soon.

Access to healthcare in general is viewed as a social responsibility. It is the ability of a person to procure specifically appropriate care when needed and sought. This may apply to Medicare patients or to patient populations at large. For access to develop into actual care there need to be adequate physician supply [with accepted assignments in case of Medicare], and financial means such as insurance or coinsurance coverage. Thus, access to care becomes actual care by way of procurement and utilization of the various dimensions of care services themselves, such as physician office visits and hospital admissions. However, even if access is somehow identified, measured and monitored its interpretation at various levels of the care process itself may vary among various socio-economic groups and regionally. For instance while there may not be any difference between blacks and whites in the Medicare program in terms of hospital discharges, some differences were found between these groups in favor of whites in terms of the rate at which some surgical procedures [e.g. open heart procedures, or hip replacement] are performed upon them, perhaps because blacks were not referred to these surgical procedures by gateway physicians as frequently as whites have been[10]. In other words, there may be some access, and care procurement, at an early stage of the care process, however, similar access for the same person may lack at a later stage of the same care process. This may be labeled as "partial/incomplete access" to care, and, therefore, what we normally refer to simply as "access to care" must imply complete access rather than partial access, for the latter may not generate the desired beneficial outcome for the patients health status, although it does contribute to healthcare costs. Furthermore, complete access may be mitigated by various factors such as the severity and urgency of the need for specialized procedures or even the patient's outlook. Consequently, what would otherwise be a *partial access* may properly be viewed as *complete access* if either the application of a foregone further procedures is not likely to improve on the patient's health status, or if the patient refuses to pursue the matter beyond the ambulatory stage of the care process. At any rate, these issues further complicate measurements and the process of monitoring access to specific care items.

This dilemma is at least partially mitigated by HCFA's decision to monitor care for Medicare beneficiaries in terms of broader rather specific dimensions. These dimensions include frequency of ambulatory visits, the proportion of people with reported health problems not receiving care, utilization of preventive care, the frequency of hospital admissions for patients who could effectively be treated in ambulatory settings, the frequency of so called referral sensitive procedures, i.e. surgical procedures which come about directly as a result of the discretionary judgment and decision of the primary care physician. The segments of the Medicare beneficiary population which are particularly subjected to access and utilization monitoring are the so called "vulnerable subgroups", i.e. people who may be subjected to barriers to care for income, socio-economic, racial, health status, and other reasons. These include those living under the poverty level, those who are eligible for both Medicare and Medicaid, without supplemental health insurance, rural populations or areas suffering from shortage of providers, and people whose available care may be curtailed by providers due to substantial fee/income cuts under the physician payment reforms.

HCFA's *1994 Report to Congress* addressed three major target issues with respect to the payment reforms: (1) anticipated income redistribution among specialities, and income diversion toward cognitive and evaluative services from the various specialities; (2) possible negative fall-out from the reforms by way of new or expanded barriers to care for the vulnerable segments of the Medicare population; and (3) impact on physician practice patterns. Some income [total billings by physicians including Part B reimbursements] appears to have been redistributed between 1991 and 1992 from surgical specialities to primary care. Specifically, allowed charges in primary care increased 13%, in some medical specialities also increased by 3%, while in the surgical specialities decreased by 4%. Preliminary data for 1993 available at the issue date of the 1994 Report suggested that the redistribution trend was to continue into that year, and will most likely be confirmed by the 1995 Report, not available at the time of this writing. There has also been an approximately 10% decline in the proportion of Part B charges attributable to inpatient care, probably reflecting the payment shift away from surgical [largely inpatient] procedures indicated earlier and a trend of reduced inpatient utilization in general in favor of more ambulatory settings, also precipitated by the Medicare prospective [DRG] hospital payment system.

The appearance of new or expanded barriers to access were assessed in terms of five criteria: frequency of ambulatory visits, the proportion of those with health problems not receiving care, preventive care utilization, frequency of hospitalization for ambulatory type conditions, and the rate of procedure performance pursuant to referrals. The elderly patient population was not found to encounter increased barriers to care, nor has the difference between whites and blacks, which may have been due to race or socio-economic status or both, in terms of ambulatory visit frequencies increased from the pre-MFS era. No significant change in access was noted geographically between 1991 and 1992, with the highest ambulatory visits continued in metropolitan areas, and the lowest in non-metropolitan areas. A smaller proportion of persons, both in the aged and the disabled categories, reported health problems without obtaining care. In fact, there were indications that patient perceived care quality, access, and costs have increased during 1992. Preventive care utilization does not seem to have improved significantly in 1992 in spite of Medicare's coverage for the elderly and the disabled. Finally, so called ambulatory care sensitive conditions, those that are treatable in ambulatory settings instead of in hospitals unless the former is not available in adequate supply, were examined to measure barriers to access to ambulatory care. Whenever and wherever the rate of hospitalization for these conditions increases, it may be seen as evidence for inadequate or insufficient ambulatory care. The Report examined 24 medical conditions in this connection for vulnerable groups, however, for 1991 only, concentrating on differences among various segments of the Medicare beneficiary population instead of the impact of the payment reform in this regard, hence changes for 1992, or 1993. Although the Report did find that some procedures emanating from referral sensitive conditions increased somewhat faster for blacks than whites, reducing historical disparities in this regard.

The payment reform's impact on physician practice patterns so far does not indicate clear trends in any desired direction, perhaps to the contrary. The two ongoing studies of a sample of Medicare patient treating physicians suggest that the average caseload of primary care physicians increased by 4-5%, for various medical specialities by up to 13%, in the historically targeted specialities of anesthesiology and radiology 8-9%, and in various areas of surgeries up to 11%, with cardiac and urological procedures having experienced the largest increases. If one expects from the payment reforms that the income redistribution aimed in favor of primary care providers and away from the specialities and in particular on the expense of surgical areas would in some way and for some reasons also alter the pattern of patient flows among these care categories, the data so far (up to 1992) does not seem to confirm that. This may be due to income-compensating provider reactions. On the other hand, while there does not so far appear to be a significant impact on practice patterns in terms of patient flows and rendered service distributions, there does seem to be a clear impact on the physicians' "average allowed charge" (AAC: Medicare reimbursement plus excess billing) by specialities between 1991-92. These charges have increased by 10% for primary care practitioners, declined for some but increased for most medical specialities, and declined for all surgical specialities in the range of 2-13%, with cardiac and general surgery experiencing the largest declines. As to income compensating service volume adjustments, a 1989 US Government study suggested that in general physicians encountering reimbursed fee reductions will compensate by increasing volume, and thereby recoup some 50% of income that would have otherwise been lost due to fee reduction[11]. Another recent study attempted to assess in connection with specific surgical procedures whether or how physicians may react to the payment adjustments by various income-compensating maneuvers, mainly by way of altering their service volume, so as to offset likely income reductions due to negative fee changes brought about by this and previous reforms. The study focused on six surgical procedure groups of which only two suggested significant compensating volume adjustments due to fee reductions[12]. Thus, income compensating volume adjustments by physicians may not be as readily implemented as physicians would perhaps desire, due mainly to increased competition in healthcare markets and, in particular, to the increasingly pervasive impact of managed care environments in these markets.

In order to assess care quality under the new Medicare physician payment system, it may be helpful to note that physicians typically receive only some fraction of what they would receive by caring for non-Medicare patients. In fact, nationally and for all services, physicians caring for Medicare beneficiaries receive only about 76% of what they would receive by caring for private, non-Medicare, patients. This ratio varies by type of service, ranging from 45% for diagnostic tests, about 51-52% for major and ambulatory surgical procedures, 71% for imaging procedures, to 92% for cognitive visit services in family practice settings. Similar variations may be noted by service category on a regional basis, where the MFS/private fee ratios range from well over 100 in rural areas to about 60% in major socially, economically or otherwise favored metropolitan areas such as Manhattan or Miami, reflecting on a greater range of geographical variations in private service fees than those suggested by the MFS. These ratios indicate the payment reform's intent to emphasize family practice in contrast to surgical procedures and diagnostic tests, and in favor of rural rather than major metropolitan areas[13].

At this point, and given the indicated ratios, one may query regarding the extent to which physician payment systems propagated by Medicare's MFS has or will spread to the care of non-Medicare beneficiaries. In other words, to what extent have non-Medicare payers emulated or will likely emulate Medicare's RBRVS/MFS fee structures? A recent study attempted to provide an answer to this question by way of a survey involving some 2,000 payers, which included HMOs, PPOs, BC/BS institutions, state Medicaid programs, as well as self-insured employers[14]. An approximately 15% response rate suggested that Medicare's payment system has spread to non-Medicare environments, although the spread is by no means uniform among the adopters, and the degree of adoption as well as applications vary among the respondents. In some cases the adoption involved only one product line while in others all product lines were involved. Thus, for instance, the Arizona Medicaid program pays MFS fees for those not in managed care plans. In general, some 17% of those surveyed implemented an RBRVS based payment system, some 40% still have it under consideration, others have either decided not to adopt, have it under development, or have not even considered it. The system is most popular among BC/BS organizations with an almost 80% adoption rate, followed by HMOs, excluding staff model ones with salaried physicians (50%), and PPOs (38%). In the public sector, 16 Medicaid programs have adopted the payment system completely, while four have partially applied it, and eleven others were considering it. The most widespread reasons for adoptions included the desire to equalize physician payments and in particular to induce primary care, to control healthcare costs, and to be compatible with the Medicare program. Given the relatively recent implementation of the Medicare payment system, even this degree of penetration appears to be impressive, and with the continuing proliferation of managed care systems along with their apparent proclivity to adopt the RBRVS-based payments, further penetration of the new Medicare physician payment mechanism into the private sector is likely. Since managed care systems tend to increase practice size, one may query the impact of practice size upon care quality.

Physician Practice Size and Care Quality

The organizational environment in which physicians practice has gone through profound changes over the years, typically from the traditional sole proprietorship to more complex institutional and group structures. Competition in the medical market place has reached an intensity never witnessed before in medical history. The supply of physicians has been steadily increasing. Physicians' traditional income levels have come to be threatened. Various ambulatory services invaded the turf of the traditional solo practitioner. Rivalry for patients increased, and the attainment of some satisfactory contract with third party payers became a worthy target, although once again a keenly competed one. Ultimately, physicians in many areas of practice were compelled to work together instead of against each other. Various organized and group practices were formed to secure a steady flow of patients as well as a reliable and continuous source of income, and resources for appropriate management. While competition in terms of price is certainly a prevalent market phenomenon, competition by way of quality imaging has become a mainstay for success. Specialization became a trademark of more intensive training hence presumably better quality care, as well as a source for organized medical practice, and multi-speciality groups have stabilized and secured desirable patient flow patterns[15]. Furthermore, the emergence of technically complex and financially very expensive diagnostic and therapeutic equipment necessitated major capital investment and commensurate management skills made possible only by larger medical practice entities and institutions. Much of this development was facilitated by the increasing preponderance of profit motivated providers in the healthcare field which have become a major source for necessary capital for themselves, and for other nonprofit major healthcare entities as well as university-based medical and research centers which have with increasing frequency sought financial and management collaboration with profit motivated entities[16]. Perennial cost containment efforts gave rise to various forms of managed care organizations with their own practice style and forms of interaction with independent providers when that happens to be the case. Medical malpractice litigation risks implanted various so called risk management programs in medical provider institutions.

The structural evolution of medical practice organizations, in particular their increasing size and complexity, is likely to have an important impact on the quality of healthcare they provide. In addition, as these organizations become larger, publicly owned, and increasingly profit motivated, conflicts and consequent trade-offs may be perceived between the organizations' financial and management interests on the one hand and the maintenance of quality in healthcare delivery on the other. Care quality and profit motives might conflict. Management's personal interests and own utility maximization efforts may be protected only on the expense of care quality delivered to the patient. Yet, larger care delivery organizations may generate positive quality outcomes. First, larger organizations are likely to have the necessary pool of financial resources for implementing effective quality assurance programs supported by sophisticated computer technology and care management talent, allowing physicians to concentrate on the quality of their practice hence providing better care, other factors and determinants relevant to care quality remaining constant[17]. Second, service volumes in specific lines of care are likely to increase with the size of the provider's organization. Furthermore, some studies have shown that care quality in a line of service is likely to increase with the volume of care items performed in that line of care service. This has particularly been shown in relation to various surgical procedures, although the positive relationship between volume and quality may not equally apply to primary care service items. Additionally, it is not always clear whether a better quality of care is due to sheer volume or to the increased concentration of human and technological resources which that volume necessitates and brings together, for in the latter case volume may be seen merely as an indirect cause of quality improvement. In fact, high volume may have a direct negative impact on care quality if it causes physicians to spread themselves thin among their patients, not pay adequate attention to individual cases, and otherwise interfere with the performance of the interpersonal components of care, discussed earlier in the volume[18].

Size may also impact quality through implementation of management that size itself often mandates. Large healthcare organizations normally have risk management and quality assurance programs, often combined. In some cases, however, the motive for and to an extent the implementation of quality control through these programs may be seen as better serving the avoidance of medical malpractice suits than pursuing quality for patient welfare concerns, although clearly the two cannot functionally and completely be separated. In most cases, what may keep the provider out of malpractice litigation may also serve the patient's welfare, particularly if medical records and charts are properly kept. At any rate, even quality assurance programs alone, without having been merged with risk management efforts, have not always been found to positively impact on quality if implemented strictly at the administrative level without active physician involvement at the local level. Nevertheless, the policy and practice standards which larger organizations often implement and enforce by way of peer and administrative oversight as well as institutionally implemented disciplinary procedures may impact positively on care quality, provided that individual patient needs are viewed as equally important inputs into clinical decisions[19]. Practice and medical records in the offices of solo practitioners normally remain within the confines of that office. Quality scrutiny is less likely, although interpersonal relationships for whatever substantive contributions they may have for care quality might be better, subject to the patient volume and practice pattern of the provider. In larger organizations, the same records are likely to be reviewed by medical peers, administrators, quality assurance personnel, and even in-house lawyers if potential legal exposure is suspected, while interpersonal relationships between provider and patient may be compromised. The trade-offs are clear, however, from a strictly technical point of view regarding the substantive quality of care as paramount, the potential for larger organizations may be more promising. Of course, these remarks must be considered in view of the complex relationships among the various components of care quality, the most important of which perhaps being the outcome dimensions of care, much of which has been discussed earlier in the volume.

Economic and Policy Functions of HCFA Databases and Files[20]

The daily maintenance and operation of the Medicare and Medicaid programs makes it necessary for HFCA to process, adjudicate and pay upon claims for healthcare cost reimbursements in accordance with various guidelines, schedules and rules. The performance of these functions is facilitated by the existence and maintenance of data and records regarding program participants, services rendered, and payments made, and these massive databases and files also make it possible for HCFA to continuously oversee, research and evaluate existing programs and their implementation. These databases and their files are maintained in three categories: (A) reference/resource data, (B) files available for utilization by the public, and (C) files for HCFA's internal consumption only. The file system is elaborate, at times complex and in terms of volume it is a giant. The rest of this chapter will briefly review parts of this extraordinarily complex system of files which are also available to the public.

The *Reference/Resource* database contains eighteen (plus a zipcode directory) utility files on various standards, coding systems and indexes. Within this group, so-called *payment policy files* are used to set Medicare reimbursement rates, with the rest containing various reference information. A few of these are reviewed here. The *adjusted average per capita cost (AAPCC) rates* file contains per capita Medicare reimbursement rates applicable to risk-based HMOs by county and reflect adjustments for age, sex, Medicare status and institutional status of Medicare beneficiaries in any given county. The *Diagnosis Related Group* (DRG) file has the DRG codes and a patient classification system, indicating patient treatment costs by hospital. The *Geographic Practice Cost Index* (GPCI) file involves all locations served by Medicare and is utilized in connection with the relative value units (RVU) along with the conversion factor to calculate Part B reimbursements under the MFS. GPCIs relate the local cost of a specific service to the national average cost for the same service and they are used to adjust national RVUs for local cost conditions. A specific GPCI is calculated for each locality and for each RVU component for that locality, that is, for physician work, practice overhead expenses, and malpractice expenses. HCFA's coding system for all procedures and services provided for Medicare beneficiaries is contained in the *Common Procedure Coding System* file which groups the codes into essentially three separate groups: the AMA's CPT-4 procedure codes, standardized HCFA codes, and local carrier specific codes. The *Medicare case-mix index* file is organized by provider number, and contains indexes which measure the cost of cases treated by specific hospitals in relation to the relevant national average. Finally, in this category, The *Relative Value Units (RVUs) of the Medicare Physician Fee Schedule* file should be noted as it contains measures of relative resource costs under the Medicare MFS and is used along with the GPCIs and a conversion factor to compute payments for various services under MFS.

Public Use Datafiles lack information which identify individuals and are used mainly by government contractors, academic researchers, and businesses which profit by reselling these data in various forms. This databank contains several file categories. The **Utilization Institutional Provider** file group contains at the present time six files. The *Hospital Service Area* file is based on inpatient claims data. Classified by provider number and zip codes, the file contains the number of discharges, average length of stay and total charges. The *Medicare Provider Analysis and Review* file (which includes the Nursing Facility and separately National Hospital files) contains data on Medicare inpatients and those also utilized skilled nursing facility. Both the hospitals and the nursing facilities are identified by unique billing numbers. The *Part B Data: Physicians, Ambulatory, Surgical Centers, and Supplier* file group of seven very useful files contain data on procedures, unidentified beneficiaries, physicians, physician fees, and medical equipment suppliers. The *Procedure* file is essentially a log of Part B procedures performed along with associated charges, while the *Beneficiary* file extracts information from claims filed by some 5% of several disadvantaged groups of beneficiaries. Four files contain data on physician participation in several dimensions. The *Physician Sample* file is based on claims information for state-based samples of Part B providers. The *National Physician Fee Schedule Relative Value* file surveys physician services by fee schedules where each record contains a procedure code, related RVUs, fee schedule coverage and payment policy codes, and related items. The *Annual Physician Fee Schedule Transition - National* file and its subset the *Carrier* files contain locality-specific pricing data under MFS for individual providers and third-party payers, where each record includes a variety of payment and pricing information and service-specific RVUs.

The *Financial Data* group of files contains nine component file sets. The *HCFA Hospital Wage Index Survey* files contain hospital hours and salaries used as inputs for DRGs. A subset of the files in this group relate to Medicare's Prospective Payment System (PPS) and contains cost as well as other statistical data utilized in setting DRGs and establishing cost limits. It covers various institutional sectors such as skilled nursing facilities, home health agencies, Part B hospital cost and charges, including capital costs. The actual computation of DRG payments utilizes the *Institutional Provider Identification and Certification* group of files, and contain records for all PPS-eligible hospitals. Similar though less detailed and more function-specific groups of datafile are set up and utilized in connection with the administration of the Medicaid program. Finally, it may be noted that most of the files are available only for mainframe processing, although many are also structured for PC users.

Notes

1.   Seplaki, L., *Cost and Competition in American Medicine: Theory, Policy and Institutions*, University Press of America, Lanham, MD, 1994, Ch 15, see in particular pp. 210-213.

2. Newhouse, J.P., Manning, W.G. et al., "Some Interim Results from a Controlled Trial of Cost Sharing in Health Insurance", *New England Journal of Medicine,* Vol. 305, 1981.
3. Pauly, M.V., *Doctors and Their Workshops: Economic Models of Physician Behavior,* University of Chicago Press, Chicago, IL, 1980. Also see, Pauly, M.V., "What is Necessary Surgery?", *Millbank Memorial Fund Quartely,* Vol. 57, 1979.
4. These and related issues were discussed in a decade of pertinent although now somewhat dated literature in Donabedian, A., *Explorations in Quality Assessment and Monitoring: The Definition of Quality and Approaches to Its Assessment* [Vol. I], *The Criteria and Standards of Quality* [Vol. II], *The Methods and Findings of Quality Assessment and Monitoring: An Illustrated Analysis* [Vol. III], Health Administration Press, Ann Arbor, MI, 1980, 1982, 1985 respectively. Donabedian, A., Wheeler, J.R.C., Wyszewianski, L., "Quality, Cost and Health: An Integrative Model", *Medical Care,* Vol. 20, 1982. Hornbrook, M.C., Berki, S.E., "Practice Mode and Payment Method: Effects on Use, Costs, Quality and Access", *Medical Care,* Vol. 23, 1985. Wennberg, J.E., Gittelsohn, A., "Variations in Medical Care in Small Areas", *Scientific American,* Vol. 246, 1982. Hadley, J., "How Should Medicare Pay Physicians?", *Milbank Memorial Fund,* Vol. 62, 1984. Wyszewianski, L., Wheeler, J.R.C., Donabedian, A., "Market-Oriented Cost-Containment Strategies and Quality of Care", *Milbank Memorial Fund,* Vol. 60, 1982.
5. Hsiao, W.C. and Stason, W.B., "Toward Developing a Relative Value Scale for Medical and Surgical Services", *Health Care Finance Review,* Vol. 1979. Gabel, J.R. and Redisch, M.A., "Alternative Physician Payment Methods: Incentives, Efficiency, and National Health Insurance", *Milbank Memorial Fund Quarterly,* Vol. 57, 1979. Jencks, S.F. and Dobson, A., "Strategies for Reforming Medicare Physician Payments: Physician Diagnosis Related Groups and Other Approaches", *New England Journal of Medicine,* Vol. 312, 1985. Roe, B., "The UCR Boondoggle: A Death Knell for Private Practice?", *New England Journal of Medicine,* Vol. 305, 1981. Burney, I.L., Schieber, G.J. et al., "Medicare and Medicaid Physician Payment Incentives", *Health Care Financing Review,* Summer 1979, and Burney, I.L., Hickman et al., "Medicare Physician Payment, Participation and Reform", *Health Affairs,* Vol. 3, 1984.
6. See Seplaki, "Supply Creates its Own Demand: Fact or Fiction", p. 200.
7. Morehead, M.A., Quality of Medical Care Provided by Family Physicians as Related to their Education, Training and Method of Practice, Health Insurance Plan of Greater New York, NY, 1958. Peterson, O.L., Andrew, L.P. et al., "An Analytical Study of North Carolina General Practice, 1953-54", *Journal of Medical Education,* Vol. 31, Part 2, 1956. For recent opinions see, Payne, B.C., Lyons, T.F. et al., *The Quality of Medical Care: Evaluation and Improvement,* Hospital Research and Educational Trust, Chicago, IL, 1976. Payne, B.C., Lyons, T.F. and Neuhaus, E., "Relationship of Physician Characteristics to Performance Quality and Improvement", *Health Services Research,* Vol.19, 1984. Rhee, S., "Factors Determining the Quality of Physician Performance in Patient Care", *Medical Care,* Vol. 14, 1976. Rhee, S., Luke, R.D. et al., "Domain of Practice and the Quality of Physician Performance", *Medical Care,* Vol. 19, 1981.
8. Federal Register, *Fee Schedule for Physicians' Services. Final Rule,* Vol. 56, No. 227, 59502-59819, Office of the Federal Register, National Archives and Records Administration, US Government Printing Office, November 25, 1991. Hsiao, W.C., Braun, P. et al., "Estimating Physicians' Work for a Resource-Based Relative Value Scale", *New England Journal of Medicine,* Vol. 319, 1988. Hsiao, W.C., Braun, P. et al., "An Overview of the Development and Refinement of the Resource-Based

Relative Value Scale", *Medical Care,* Vol. 30 (Supp.), November 1992. Physician Payment Review Commission, *Annual Report to Congress, 1989,* US Government Printing Office, Washington, DC, 1989. See also, a brief historical recount in Seplaki, cited in Note #1, pp. 204-206. The various issues and available options considered by Congress are recounted in Ginsburg, P.B., "Physician Payment Policy in the 101st Congress", *Health Affairs,* Vol. 8, Spring 1989.

9.   Health Care Financing Administration, *1991 Annual Report to Congress: Moni-toring Changes in Use of, Access to, and Appropriateness of Part B Medicare Ser-vices,* Office of Research and Demonstrations, Baltimore, MD, May 2, 1991. Health Care Financing Administration, *1992 Annual Report to Congress: Monitoring Utilization of, and Access to Services for Medicare Beneficiaries Under Part B Medicare Services. Physician Payment Reform,* Office of Research and Demonstra-tions, Baltimore, MD, May 21, 1992. Health Care Financing Administration, *Third Annual Report to Congress: Monitoring Utilization of, and Access to Services for Medicare Beneficiaries Under Physician Payment Reform,* Office of Research and Demonstrations, Baltimore, MD, May 6, 1993. Report to Congress: Monitoring The Impact of Medicare Payment Reform on Utilization and Access, HCFA Pub. No. 03358, Office of Research and Demonstrations, Baltimore, MD, September 1994. See also, HCFA, Special Report, Vol. 2, *Hospital Data by Geographic Area for Aged Medicare Beneficiaries: Selected Procedures, 1986,* HCFA Pub. No. 03300. Office of Research and Demonstrations, US Printing Office, Washington, DC, 1990, and HCFA, Special Report, Vol. 3, *Rehospitalization by Geographic Area for Aged Medicare Beneficiaries: Selected Procedures, 1986-87,* HCFA Pub. No. 03303, US Printing Office, Washington, DC, 1990.

10.   Millman, M. (ed.), *Access to Health Care In America,* Institute of Medicine, Com-mittee on Monitoring Access to Personal Health Care Services, National Academic of Sciences, National Academy Press, Washington, DC, 1993. Cited in HFCA 1994, *Annual Report to Congress.*

11.   US Congressional Budget Office, *Volume Responses to Exogenous Changes in Medicare's Payment Rates,* Technical memorandum, August 1989.

12.   Lee, J.A., Mitchell, J.B., "Physician Reaction to Price Changes: An Episode-of-Care Analysis", *Health Care Financing Review,* Vol. 16, No. 2, Winter 1994.

13.   Miller, M.E., Zuckerman, S. and Gates, M., "How Do Medicare Physician Fees Compare With Private Payers?", *Health Care Financing Review,* Vol. 14, No. 3, Spring 1993. Pope, G.C., Cromwell, J. et al., *A Comparison of Medicare Physician Fees, Physician Charges, Fees of Other Payors, and Model Medical Fee Schedule Amounts,* Cooperative Agreement #99-C-99256/1-06, Center for Health Economics Research, Waltham, MA, July 1991.

14.   McCormack, L.A., Burge. RT., "Diffusion of Medicare RBRVS and Relayed Payment Policies", *Health Care Financing Review,* Vol. 16, No. 2, Winter 1994. This article also discussed the formula utilized for physician fee determination.

15.   Ludmerer, K.M., *Learning to Heal: The Development of American Medical Educa-tion,* Basic Books, New York, 1985. Stevens, R., *American Medicine and the Public Interest,* Yale University Press, New Haven, CT, 1971. See also Nash, D.B. (ed.), *Future Practice Alternatives in Medicine,* Igaku-Shoin, New York, 1987; Ottensmeyer, D.J. and Smith, H.L., "Patterns of Medical Practice in an Era of Change", *Frontiers of Health Service Management,* 1986, and Ginzberg, E., "The Destabilization of Health Care", *New England Journal of Medicine,* Vol. 315, 1986.

16.   Reinhardt, U., "Financial Capital and Healthcare Growth Trends" in Gray, B.H. (ed.), *For Profit Enterprise in Health Care,* National Academy Press, Washington, DC, 1986. Light, D.W., "Corporate Medicine for Profit", *Scientific American,* Vol.

6, 1986, and Johnson, R.L., "The Myth of Dominance by National Health Care Corporations", *Frontiers of Health Service Management*, Vol. 1986.

17. McCabe, O.P., "Physician Response to Computer Reminders", *JAMA*, Vol. 244, 1980. Thompson, M.S. et al., "Resource Requirements for Evaluating Ambulatory Health Care", *American Journal of Public Health*, Vol. 74, 1984. Thompson, M.S. et al., "The Cost of Quality Assurance in Medicine", *Evaluations in the Health Professions*, Vol. 6, 1983. Friedman, R.H., "The Use of Computers to Assist Physicians in Patient Management", *Advances in Internal Medicine*, Vol. 31, 1986.

18. Donabedian, A., "Volume, Quality and the Regionalization of Health Care Services", *Medical Care*, Vol. 22, 1984. Flood, A.B., Scott, W.R., Ervy, W., "Does Practice Make Perfect?", *Medical Care*, Vol. 22, 1984. Luft, H.S., "The Relationship Between Surgical Volume and Mortality", *Medical Care*, Vol. 18, 1980.

19. Eddy, D.M., "Clinical Policies and the Quality of Clinical Practice", *New England Journal of Medicine*, Vol. 307, 1982. See also, Pena, J.J., Pena, B.M. and Rosen, B., "Combining Risk Management and Quality Assurance" in Pena, J.J., Haffner, A.N. et al. (eds), *Hospital Quality Assurance*, Aspen Publications, Rockville, MD, 1984. Deuschle, J.M. et al., "Physician Performance in a PrePaid Heal Plan", *Medical Care*, Vol. 20, 1982. Palmer, R.H. et al., "A Randomized Trial of Quality Assurance in Sixteen Ambulatory Care Practices", *Medical Care*, Vol. 23, 1985, and by the same author "Does Quality Assurance Improve Ambulatory Care?", *Journal of Ambulatory Care Management*, Vol. 4, 1986.

20. This material is based on *Overview of Health Care Financing Administration Data: Resource Guide*, and internal document prepared by HCFA/BDMS/OHCIS/ILB, March 1995.

8 Cost–Quality Relationships

Some years ago a patient entered a California hospital with back and leg problems not knowing that her case may turn out to be the first judicial consideration of the tradeoff between cost containment by way of utilization review and medical malpractice liability. Medi-Cal, California's assistance program, was to cover her cost. Since after the operations her recovery was slower than anticipated, the patient's physician requested authority from Medi-Cal to extend her stay in the hospital. Authority was granted for only about half of the requested extension. After having been discharged from the hospital, the patient developed clotting and an infection. Upon readmission a few days later, her leg had to be amputated. During the ensuing litigation, the patient's medical expert testified that her leg could have been saved if she had not been prematurely discharged. After a jury award of a half-million dollars in the lower court, the California Court of Appeals reversed judgment finding that the patient's discharge was consistent with applicable standards of care, and even the patient's own physician did not object to the early discharge at the time that it was being implemented. While holding Medi-Cal not liable, the court did state, however, that in general patients may recover for damages in cases where needed care was denied even if due to nationally recognized cost containment efforts[1]. This case may have also set the stage for the various legal issues related to care quality and cost containment, issues which will be dealt with in the latter chapters of the volume. At this stage, we will take a closer look at the economic and social policy issues involved, and at some of the underlying causes and sources of the cost-quality tradeoff.

Many of the underlying reasons for the current preoccupation with cost-quality tradeoffs emanate from recent and more distant past developments on the American healthcare scene. Containing healthcare expenditures, and in particular the rate of increase in healthcare expenditures, has become a matter of public policy. Labor, employers, government, beneficiary groups and third-party payers have individually and sometimes in coordination set out to achieve cost containment goals. On the other hand, there is not enough evidence to indicate that these forces are prepared to compromise by a way of similar reductions in the volume and perhaps nature of medical services rendered to individual patients so as to achieve cost containment. The cause of cost containment is socially and politically mandated while corresponding reductions in the volume and perhaps the nature of care are viewed as likely sources for care quality compromises. These apparent contradictions are played out in an environment where constantly improving and evolving high cost medical technology is not only applied but is also demanded in the name of diagnostic and therapeutic care quality, and are utilized in settings outside the traditional hospital, such as ambulatory surgical, MRI, and cardiac catheterization centers. These not only raise issues of cost but also quality within free-standing clinical environments, a matter discussed earlier in the volume.

Then there is the "marketization" of medicine. It is believed that participants in competitive medical markets strive for decreasing costs, sustain desirable financial performance for all ownership groups whether private or public, and at the same time maintain adequate supply of necessary care. Marketization directly and indirectly causes integration in the industry giving birth to large managed care organizations. Providers merge with insurance carriers, providers sustain self-insurance, insurers and third-party payers provide healthcare, so much so that the traditional lines of demarcation between insurer and provider has almost disappeared. All this generates a confusing melting-pot in medicine where costs are supposed to be constrained, but services are to remain on standard, new technology is to be applied when and where needed, and competition among providers is supposed to dominate. Large individual or well organized independent purchasers of healthcare services use or coordinate purchasing power aimed at reducing their healthcare cost at some acceptable level of quality. Physicians and institutional providers compete for patients in terms of care costs, technologically advanced facilities, and care quality.

In spite of these efforts, while the rate of growth in healthcare costs has been somewhat lowered during recent years, healthcare costs have not decreased. The quantity of care services dispensed continues to increase, and as we noted earlier there is considerable uncertainty as to whether or not quality has suffered in the various environments where healthcare is delivered. The problem appears to be imbedded in the relationship between healthcare quality and costs. Costs are often difficult to reduce without reducing at least the volume of services. Yet, a reduction in the volume of services is often perceived as a reduction in the quality of care, although it need not always be the case. In addition, risk management programs designed to reduce the likelihood of malpractice liability tend to suggest that if the quality impact of a procedure is not certain then do it rather than go without it so as to avoid later assertions that not having performed a procedure in fact caused the problem and that had the procedure been performed or performed on time (in case of administrative delays) the source of liability could have been averted.

The balancing act between cost containment and the maintenance of some desired or desirable quality standards is a very delicate one. The delicacy is made more complex by data quality and measurement disparities. Measuring cost is usually a relatively easy accounting or administrative task. The data is explicit and normally readily available. Measuring quality, as we have seen earlier in this volume is quite a different story. Even if properly and functionally defined, quality may be very difficult to measure under a variety of care environments. Given inadequate information and data bases, may be difficult to ascertain whether quality has been reduced or enhanced by virtue of having or not having undertaken a care transaction. Related to this dilemma is the degree of improvement in health status which is needed to consider as adequate or even desirable for an improvement in healthcare quality. In other words, what is the value of the care to patient, particularly if the improvement in healthcare status is only marginal, and short-term? What standards are there to determine what term is too short, and for who? Once again, the care cost-quality balancing act is very delicate, even if its nature and perceived function is clearly identified, and much written about. This chapter will examine in detail the nature and some of the dimensions of these socio-economic acrobatics.

The Cost-Quality Dichotomy: A Review of Some Findings

The precise answer to the question regarding the extent to which healthcare costs can be cut without significantly compromising care quality has yet to be formulated by anyone. It is understood, however, that one way to reduce costs without compromising quality is by increasing the efficiency of the care process. But how much efficiency is left in the system? It is quite possible that past cost-containment measures such as Medicare's Prospective Payment System and private initiatives may have already extracted much of whatever inefficiencies the system may have harbored. This does not mean that until the past fifteen years or so when cost control efforts have really gained momentum there was no preoccupation with the trade-off dilemma between costs and quality. In fact, hospital care quality has been a significant variable in several past studies of a microeconomic nature aimed at scrutinizing hospital management decisions under rational constraints. Some twenty-five years ago, at least one study has made hospital management utility a function of both the quality and quantity of care provided at the hospital. Higher patient census and higher care quality, mostly in structural and process terms, were seen as determinants of the level of hospital management utility[2]. Another early study made hospital quality, as perceived by the hospital, a function of the number of employees per patient day and the volume of supplies. Costs were determined by input volume and price, and an increase in the number of employees and supplies always assumed to yield a positive incremental change in healthcare quality. The study's later version emphasized healthcare quality in a more marketable context, namely quality as perceived by the patient and his/her physician. It, once again, found a positive relationship between structural and process increments in care and corresponding changes in health status[3]. In other words, improvements in care quality necessitated additional resources, or putting it still another way, higher care quality meant higher costs and, importantly, vice versa. These theses suggest that care quality must yield to cost containment so that as costs are contained care quality is reduced.

Cost and care quality, however, have not always been seen as moving together. Some studies from the early 1980s suggest that throwing more money at the process will not always yield higher quality, in fact at some point and at least theoretically there may be negative relationships[4]. The theories rest on the notion of an "ideal physician" - a practitioner who chooses and applies resources available to him or her in a most efficient manner so as to attain a targeted maximum improvement in the patient's health status, subject to medical state of the art constraints. This model assumes an optimum relationship among care cost, care quality and provider efficiency (care strategy), a relationship which is relevant only to the "ideal physician". "Sub-ideal physicians" may apply more resources with inadequate care strategy and efficiency hence experience a deterioration in the patient's health status in spite of the greater cost. Thus, in reality, the outcome of care cannot be predicted by simply measuring the level or increment in costs without observing associated efficiency and applied competence. The role and functional performance of the physician becomes an integral part of the cost-quality relationship.

Theoretical relationships between healthcare cost and quality are obviously unclear. Based on a number of studies, so are the empirical relationships. Let us take a brief look at a number of relevant studies. A relatively recent study suggests a very complex non-linear and at times inconsistent relationship between healthcare costs and quality. Reiterating its essence in general terms, the study used cost data on 657 hospitals to estimate a variable cost function, and proxied care quality by outcome in terms of risk-adjusted re-admission and mortality rates. A statistically significant relationship was found between variable costs and general re-admission rates for hospital inpatient populations. Specifically, medical and surgical re-admissions and surgical mortality proved to be statistically significant determinants of variable costs. In general, the cost-quality relations were non-linear though not monotonically increasing. In fact, within some quality ranges quality improvements were found along with negative marginal costs, i.e. cost decreases. The cost-quality relationship was fluctuating around a given average variable cost level at different levels of quality, suggesting that up to a certain point it may be possible to attain consecutively higher levels care quality with a relatively constant average cost level. Presumably a lesson for hospital administrators[5].

Complex empirical cost-quality relationship was also shown in an earlier study which contrasted the quality of care offered by Stanford medical faculty with that offered by other physicians from the community in twelve different DRGs[6]. The outcome of care was measured in terms of survival. Using logistic regression, the researchers attempted to predict the cost of care and survival rates of patients based on variables such as urgency of admission (but not case severity), DRGs, patient age and gender. Actual/predicted cost ratios and their geometric means were generated for each patient under the two care categories, i.e. faculty and community, and the geometric means were multiplied by the average cost for all patients involved in both care categories. Adjusted mortality measures were generated in the same manner. Faculty care was found to be both more costly and superior in terms of inpatient survival rates for three of the twelve DRGs. In another five DRG groups, faculty care was found to be superior in terms of mortality rates but with the same average cost level as encountered in community care settings. The other four DRG groups showed higher cost of care but no better outcomes in the faculty care environment than those experienced in community care settings. Once again, the cost-quality relationship in healthcare could not be demonstrated to be a simple linear one where quality would vary with and in some direct proportion of costs.

Another study contrasted the impact of the service's time dimension, i.e. the number of days of stay, with service intensity, i.e. the number of services performed per day of stay[7]. It is assumed that, barring free service or the unlikely event that a physician will pay for the privilege of performing a service for a patient, both an increase in the number of days of service and/or an increase in the intensity of service per day generates positive marginal costs, that is, the total cost of care will increase with an increase in both the number of days and/or the number of services performed per day. Yet, while quality appears to have improved with one, it did not improve with the other. Better outcome was found to have resulted from greater service intensity, but not from a greater number of days of stay. In fact, the relationship with respect to the latter was negative, i.e. longer stay yielded poorer results. However, the study did not control for case severity and case-mix. Thus, it is possible that longer patient stays could be associated with or caused by greater severity of illness, hence the less favorable result in terms of outcome, calling into question the causality if any that may be involved in the negative relationship between outcome and length of stay.

In addition to these, a number of other studies attempted to delineate some meaningful relationships between the cost of care and care outcome of various forms, using various methods. One such study found a positive relationship between costs and mortality rates in hospital settings, suggesting a higher death rate with higher costs, but not indicating that lower death rates would be achieved with lower expenditures. This emanates mainly from longer hospital stays caused by greater levels of case severity. The severity of hospital case-loads is likely to vary directly not only with costs but also with mortality or negative outcomes. Another study confirmed the complexity of this issue by postulating cubic relationship between cost and quality. Specifically in the lower and upper regions of the cost-quality function a positive relationship was found between the variables, while in the mid-region a negative relationship was demonstrated. The reasons for the negative relationship, that is cost varying inversely with quality, were attributed to the positive impact of experience. As volume increases proportionately fewer mistakes are made and care strategies with lower costs and higher effectiveness can be formulated using the benefits of increased experience. Two other studies found a positive relationship between cost and quality, that is higher costs seem to have yielded lower inpatient mortality rates. In all of these studies, however, the results clearly depended upon a number of factors, such as whether or not there were controls for inpatient case-severity or case-mix, the size of the hospital sample, the size and the characteristics of the hospitals included, and the extent to which the hospitals included can be viewed as representative of that service sector. At times, findings regarding healthcare cost-quality relationships were merely inciden-tal to a different primary purpose of the study which was not designed to identify cost-quality relationships in the first place[8]. It appears that the final word, if there can be such a thing, on the theoretical and empirical causal relationships between healthcare quality and healthcare cost in general and in specific care and institutional situations, and even only in hospital environ-ments, leaving out ambulatory settings for the moment, has yet to be spoken.

Healthcare cost-quality relationship may also be investigated by way of possible relationships between care quality and *profitability*. After the imple-mentation of Medicare's DRG payment system and the proliferation of managed care organizations, hospitals have increasingly found themselves in strained financial condition, not unlike other business organizations in the rest of the economy. Hospitals have closed and many have been absorbed by larger units or hospital systems. Attempting to survive in an increasingly competitive market place, total profits and profit margins have come into focus. In addition to pricing, which is now often constrained by third-party payers including the US and state governments and by coordinated purchas-ing groups with significant market power, care quality became a measure of success and instrument of provider service marketing. Quality has come into the center of attention by way of various internal programs [QA, RM, etc. discussed in Ch. 6] aimed specifically at monitoring and presumably im-proving care quality both as perceived by the provider and by the patient. However, as one may query the relationship between cost and quality, so should one wonder about the impact of a relentless drive by institutions to survive to be as profitable as possible upon the quality of care provided.

A number of studies have found the relationship between quality and profitability in industries outside the healthcare sector, particularly in manu-facturing, quite significant. In this relationship quality was seen as the cause of increased sales and market shares, or as the source of opportunity for charging a higher price even with constant sales. Increased productivity and efficiency with quicker patient recovery hence lower cost per patient stay and consequently higher profits were also traced back to care quality[9]. Indeed, hospitals performing better than others in terms of return on equity have apparently done so by way of cost controls and by increasing market shares, both of which have been identified as the links in the causation between care quality and financial performance[10].

A 1989 Health Trust study of 82 hospitals in 21 states and in various market situations was designed to throw some additional light on the rela-tionship between hospital profitability and care quality[11]. *Financial per-*

formance was measured by net operating income/net operating revenue ratios. *Quality* was depicted by way of perceptions on the part of patients, providers and others involved, and applied to overall quality and the quality of services provided by nurses and physicians. The extent to which managed care and Medicare were present in the market areas, as well as care quality, proved to be the only significant predictors of financial performance. Hospitals providing better care were found to hold higher market shares or were more efficient, or both. Variables such as population, income levels, hospital size in terms of number of beds, and competition intensity in the market areas were not found to be significant predictors of profitability. The study did not test the impact on the profitability-quality relationship of other perhaps relevant variables such as service mix, physician practice patterns, case mix, and hospital pricing patterns in the various markets.

Simple Logistics of Cost-Quality Relationships

The relationship between cost and quality may be depicted by a simple formula such as $Q_t = O_t/C_t$, where Q is the quality of medical care, O is quality demonstrated in terms of outcome, and C is the cost of that care, all during time period t. This equation may be expanded by adding other components of care quality, such as structure and process thus yielding $Q_t = O_t + S_t + P_t/C_t$. The interpretation of either formula suggests an obvious direct (positive) relationship between quality and its definitional components, holding costs constant, and an adverse (negative) relationship between cost and quality, holding outcome and its related variables constant. None of this is inconsistent with some of the studies that I have examined here, and perhaps many others that have been done which I did not discuss. Using this formula may run into measurement problems. Costs on first glance are probably not difficult to measure although even that may be at the mercy of accounting techniques utilized, records available, and the decision whether only direct costs should be considered, or indirect costs as well. Health outcome may be assessed as we have seen in terms of the patient's health status, functional status or number of life-years saved, during the time period involved. If we allow for the possibility that ultimate health status cannot be realistically measured during time period t, and that therefore the measurement needs more than one time period such as t + (t + 1), or even t + (t + 1) + (t + 2) then the initial formula becomes $Q_t = O_{t + (t + 1) + (t + 2)} /C_{t + (t + 1) + (t + 2)}$.

The notation can be significantly simplified by allowing a long enough time period in the first place for the effects of the treatment to completely work themselves out. As I reasoned in Chapters 4 and 5, that may be difficult if not impossible in many cases. However, if some time period [or a sequence of time periods where various stages of health status improvement occur] can be identified t, t + 1, and t + 2 become sub-periods of the projected total period T, where T = t + (t + 1) + (t + 2) needed for the treatment to generate a final outcome, if that time period is known, and if the "final outcome" *per se*, other than mortality, or perhaps one measured in relation to expected outcome, can readily be identified. Similar assertions in terms of time may apply to the extended formula which also includes *structure* and *process*. However, their actual measurement may be quite a different matter[12]. I will not repeat the various issues and relevant problems, discussed earlier in the volume.

A rearrangement of the initial version of the formula yields $O_t = C_t Q_t$, which may also be consistent with the results of some of the empirical studies reviewed. Specifically, if the general quality of care is held constant, an increase in costs generates an improvement in outcome which we have seen to be quite likely if, for instance, during any given hospital-day the amount of services [service intensity] is increased. This would also apply to the expanded version of the formula as well where process likely increases with cost and service intensity, while structure remains constant in any given time period(s). A further rearrangement yields $C_t = O_t / Q_t$, and the possibility that, holding outcome constant, cost varies inversely with quality. This could be the case with an overutilization of services, tests, and particularly diagnostic procedures to the point where the increased risks involved in such procedures outweigh the potential benefits, while obviously increasing costs. This conclusion would not necessarily follow to the same extent from the extended formula where increased service intensity would likely increase process, although holding structure constant would be feasible. At any rate, these algebraic manipulations which can be further extended and presented in various other forms allow us to visualize quality, cost, and outcome relationships in a clearer though rudimentary and simplified form. In fact, further thoughts may be generated in this regard by allowing for the possibility, for instance, that the variables may change in the same or opposite direction but do so at different rates. For instance, Q may decrease if C increases at a faster rate than O [or, O + S + P]. While this is less likely with some individual patients and "ideal physicians", it is quite possible throughout the healthcare system which is populated with a variety of patient and physician types. In fact, instances for this notion may not be difficult to find from the recent past. Thus, we may speak of the "social" and "private" quality of healthcare, and a difference between the quality and cost of healthcare for individuals, or even individual groups, and society as a whole. This consideration clearly has social and political relevance at a time of smoldering healthcare reform controversies.

For scholars attempting to pursue these and similar issues empirically, measurements and data become paramount. Thus, one may seek the unit of measurement in connection with healthcare services when examining their cost, quality, and importantly the tradeoffs, if any, between cost and quality. Allowing for a change in the length of a time period or a series of consecutive applicable time periods during which the characteristics of these units (even if properly defined initially) may change only compounds the complexities involved. The concern here is justified since a treatment process and structure expected to lead to a certain outcome may change, and do so several times, in the course of the total treatment period. Each such change will likely necessitate a revision of the applicable unit of measurement both for quality and for costs. Hence, it is not inconceivable that one may find different cost-quality relationships even within one single treatment process before it leads to some sort of outcome, and the "true" or overall cost-quality relationship may not be ascertained until the outcome ("final outcome" - however, that may defined) has been reached. For instance, a stroke victim might well recover to a stage, removed from the ICU, began rehabilitation treatment, various therapies, and so forth. If expected "final outcome" can be defined, it is probably sometime after the removal from the ICU and at some stage where therapies and other treatments are no longer needed or applied either because the patient has completely recovered, or because no further improvement can be expected. In either case, cost-quality tradeoffs may need to be considered at each stage of the treatment process, and, as I noted earlier, those relationships may well be different at each stage.

Furthermore, at each stage of the treatment process the units of measurements for both costs and quality are likely to change. However, the reduction in cost or an increase in quality, or both, may not always be clear. Let us illustrate the point by first using an analogy from a non-medical sector. Assume that genetic engineering produces a new kind of watermelon, the average size of which is three times a large as the average of those produced before the innovation. Query: did the cost of the melon go down or did its quality increase, or both? An answer probably rests with the way watermelons are sold. Everything else remaining equal, sale by the *weight* would imply a cost/unit reduction for the producer, while sale at a higher price by the *piece* would suggest an improvement in perceived quality if the new melons were more popular i.e. their demand curve would shift to the right. A quality improvement per unit (i.e. for each melon) occurred. What are the units of sale in healthcare? For instance, in the case of the stroke victim what is (or are) the unit(s) of measure for the initial, e.g. EMS service? What units for measurement may be attached to the services of the physicians and nurses in the ICU, the subsequent therapists, and so forth? Perhaps time weighted with a service intensity factor. If so, costs would be derived by applying some sort of monetary values for each unit [refer to the previous chapter which discussed the pricing of physicians services]. What about units of measure for quality, at each stage and overall? Can cost-quality tradeoffs be measured or even meaningfully interpreted at each stage of the entire process to "final outcome", or should it be left until the "final outcome" has been attained. It is quite likely that the nature and the direction of the relationship between cost and quality at each and every one of the process stages for the stroke victim might be different. For instance, at the crucial first few minutes, it is quite possible that quality in terms of service benefits and interim outcomes will far exceed the cost EMS service, and quality will increase with minimum or zero marginal cost. At later stages of the care, with the introduction of professional services normally recognized by many as higher caliber, such as those of nurses and physicians, quality in terms of interim benefits and positive interim outcome may vary directly and perhaps even proportionately with costs, or costs might outpace interim improvements, and do so until the anticipated "final outcome" by way of complete or substantial recovery occurs. These and many more possible questions that could be raised indicate that considerably more thought and research are needed before socially optimum policy measures may be devised that could effectively deal with complex cost-quality relationships.

The Role of Quality in Cost-Benefit/Cost-Effectiveness Analyses

We noted earlier that the relationship between healthcare cost and quality is complex and not necessarily predictable. Incurring additional costs may generate more healthcare but not necessarily better healthcare. We noted that more healthcare may come in greater intensity and/or in larger quantity. Based on the reviewed statistical studies, the former is likely to improve quality, the latter, however, may very well not. Yet, studies have also shown that on occasion increased healthcare quality may occur without additional costs and even with cost reduction if efficiencies can be exploited without compromising quality. These complex issues and inconsistencies in healthcare cost-quality relationships may have significant implications for healthcare policy. Fundamental questions would address the dilemma of what projects to undertake or expand and which ones should be cut or eliminated. In healthcare endeavors, do the benefits outweigh the costs, or vice-versa. And, if expected benefits are greater than costs, will those benefits manifest themselves in provisions for needed healthcare of adequate quality? Thus, "benefits" implies a standard level of quality, where "standard" is likely to be evaluated in terms of community values applicable to the location of the care delivery. Healthcare cost-quality issues, therefore, become a focus of relevant public policies, for the responsibility of any national healthcare policy is not only to ensure the delivery of healthcare, but also that such healthcare should be of adequate quality.

Healthcare policies are made subject to various constraints, including quality and economic. Decisions to spend moneys also involve choices among alternatives within a group of healthcare related goals. To ascertain that moneys and resources are utilized efficiently, the need for and social utility of a project is evaluated and compared to alternative projects. In principle, the expected direct and indirect benefits from a project for all concerned may exceed (but should at least equal) its direct and indirect costs for all involved. In short, if these costs and benefits (social costs and social benefits) are known $SB > SC$, i.e. the social benefits (SB) from a project should exceed (or, at least equal) its social cost (SC). Where the *marginal social benefit* (MSB) from a project is equal to the project's *marginal social cost* (MSC) a state of "social optimum" is attained and all applicable resources are said to be utilized in their most efficient manner. The task of cost-benefit analysis is to procure and apply all necessary data and information regarding a project so that a rational decision as to the undertaking of that project, aimed at a social optimum, may be reached. Since the decision needs to be made before the project begins, the assessment of the project's costs and benefits must also take place before the project actual gets underway and expressed at that time. The viability of the project thus needs to be expressed as a ratio of project benefits to project costs (B/C) at the beginning of the project, that is, both variables having been stripped of their time value for each year over the project's total life. The values are discounted over the expected life of the project. A project is expected to have a positive net benefit if $B/C > 1$, suggesting that the present (discounted) value of social benefits is greater than the present value of social costs. However, this ratio does not provide enough information for actually choosing a project, for several competing projects may have ratios greater than one, but decisively different net benefits (NB): the difference between social benefits and social costs of the project. In other words, B-C for each competing project should also be taken into consideration. In fact, some projects with higher B/C ratios may harbor lower net benefits. Finally, we should note that relying on B/C ratios, net social benefits, or both for project selection presupposes reliability of measurements, data and valuations. It also presupposes that benefits and costs relevant for the project are properly identified and not duplicated, the latter referring again to measurement problems. These may be difficult to achieve under circumstances where there may not yet be a market, hence prices for the goods and services which the project is expected to generate in the future. In fact, even if a market with a relevant price structure can be envisioned in advance of the project, the prices used to evaluate both benefits and costs are not likely to generate true and comprehensive marginal social costs and marginal social benefits if substantial monopoly powers are present in the relevant product and input markets, or if significantly measurable fallouts can be anticipated by third parties.

Beyond data identification, measurement and valuation issues for each of the years involved in some total expected life of the project, the total life of the project and the discount rate to be utilized for present value calculations need also to be established. In general, the shorter the expected project life the lower is the risk involved in the miscalculation of prices, costs and benefits, and the less likely that the currently chosen project might in some way pre-empt some future in many respects superior projects. As to interest (discount rates), and barring perfectly competitive markets where there is only one interest rate that is equal to the rate of return on capital and on private savings, various money market and capital market variables need to be considered and for different time periods. Rates generally vary directly with the length of the project and with the risks involved. If the project utilizes private undertakers' own funds, then the rate should reflect what could be earned with the funds in their best alternative utilization (opportunity cost). With social projects undertaken by a government or social agencies, the rate should again reflect an opportunity cost, i.e. what the funds could earn in their best private sector alternatives[13].

The complexities regarding cost benefit valuations we noted in the general economic sector multiply in the healthcare sector. Highly subjective variables such as human life, positive or negative changes in longevity, improvement or deteriorations in health status, and the frequently unknown time periods involved in connection with these outcomes, make reliable cost-benefit valuations even more difficult than in the non-medical sector. Further compounding the calculations is the fact that a proper treatment project today will avert additional often unknown and in view of rapidly developing technology constantly changing healthcare costs at some future date which, notwithstanding the difficulties, should also be considered in the cost-benefit balance. Some studies have attempted to measure human life using a so called human capital approach. More specifically it relies on the present value of a person's future income stream foregone due to a loss of life or permanent total injury. While it is a standard and reliable method utilized in personal injury and wrongful death cases litigated in the judiciary, and it does measure a person's lost earning capacity hence the corresponding lost portion of national output, it does not directly measure a person's ability or willingness to pay for avoiding mortality or morbidity. It is in terms of this willingness to pay that actual social welfare losses or gains have been esti-mated by some other studies[14].

An application of cost-benefit analysis in healthcare can be found in a relatively recent study which focused on tests and procedures aimed at screening for sexually transmitted diseases (STDs) in otherwise healthy women[15]. The cost side of the equation includes the explicit financial cost of the process, time spent, treatment costs, and averted future costs. Benefits were measured in terms of treatment improvement due to early detection via the tests, positive fallout from not allowing the disease to spread due to early detection, and the psychological benefits of reassurance that ensue from a negative test result. A survey of providers generated dollar values for the variables involved. This was one study that received considerable attention. However, so far there have not been many. Nevertheless, while cost-benefit analyses have not been frequently applied in the healthcare sector, probably because of notorious valuation and measurement difficulties, it or its versions have been utilized at times. Thus, comparing the benefits and risks associated with a treatment with a view to ascertaining that potential benefits exceed the risks by some unspecified but "wide" margin may be considered to be an application of the cost-benefit principle, even though it does not consider the cost of treatment inputs involved[16].

An alternative to cost-benefit analyses, *cost-effectiveness* (CES) studies are techniques for identifying the effective utilization of a given amount of resources. While originally developed by and for the military, it has become a common sight in health policy analyses. CES systematically summarize the resources utilized and the resulting health benefits expected for alternative healthcare programs in order to enable policy makers to make a choice among various policy alternatives. It is frequently applied in preventive health programs by comparing various policy efforts aimed at diseases and population segments[17].

Since they not only attempt to assign monetary values to health outcomes and treatment results, CES is simpler to implement than benefit analyses. It uses descriptive yardsticks like additional years of life procured by a treatment. CES may also aim at finding a specific program which can attain a healthcare or policy goal with the minimum amount/cost of needed resources. Thus, CES analyze the tradeoff between monetary and health effects. The major steps in the studies normally include (a) defining a program, (b) computing net costs, (c) determining net health effects in terms of additional years of life, (d) applying decision rules, and (e) performing sensitivity analyses: varying uncertain parameters, recomputing costs and health effects, and setting new decisions.

As with cost-benefit analyses, the most often encountered problem with CES is the lack of adequate data and information. While this problem often reduces the precision of CES, they can still yield considerable benefits when policy decisions need to be undertaken promptly under social and political pressures. Furthermore, in contrast to cost-benefit analyses, it does not require "monetization" and using sensitivity analyses it can better deal with data problems. Another problem may relate to incorporating consumer preferences into the analyses since lay patient responses may need to be interpreted so that they can be accommodated by the technical parameters of the model. In addition, human nature and frequently human responses and humanistic values may be far too subjective and difficult to quantify. Yet, at least an attempt may be preferred to no attempt at all for even broad results can be used as general guidelines for supporting or negating certain policy decisions.

Finally, a word on the strength of CES in the healthcare sector. The amount of resources that can be allocated to this sector has always been and will be limited. Resource constraints and cost-containment efforts will continue to force difficult decisions upon policy-makers. Various projects such as primary prevention, early detection, researching new cases or improving the treatment of old ones, and many more, all compete for a limited amount of resources. CES can be helpful in making decisions in these and other similarly broad healthcare areas because it has the framework for organizing general information regarding the effectiveness and efficiency of alternative health programs. In other words, it remains a useful policy research tool. In a more global context, however, CES as a policy-oriented research tool is probably inferior to cost-benefit analyses. The former is useful for projects which impact mainly on healthcare: CES is typically sector specific. The latter, however, can also be used for inter-sectoral studies generating results for inter-sectoral policy choices. This may be important for broader political and policy decisions at Federal, state or even local government levels where issues of allocating scarce resources among various alternatives, where the healthcare sector is only one such alternative, are often called into question.

Notes

1. Wickline v. State 228 Cal Reptr 661 (Cal. App. 2d Dist 1986). Cited in *ABA Journal,* June 1, 1988, p. 26.
2. Newhouse, J.P., "Toward a Theory of Nonprofit Institutions: An Economic Model of a Hospital", *American Economic Review,* Vol. 60, No. 1, 1970.
3. Feldstein, M.S., "Hospital Cost Inflation: A Study of Nonprofit Price Dynamics", *American Economic Review,* Vol. 61, No. 5, 1971; and Feldstein, M.S., "Quality Change and the Demand for Hospital Care", *Econometrica,* Vol. 45, No. 7, 1977.
4. Donabedian, A., *Explorations in Quality Assessment and Monitoring.* Vol. I, *The Definition of Quality and Approaches to its Assessment,* Health Administration Press, Ann Arbor, MI, 1980. Donabedian, A., Wheeler, J.R.C. and Wyszewianski, L., "Quality, Cost and Health: An Integrative Model", *Medical Care,* Vol. 20, No. 10, 1982.
5. Fleming, S.T., *Toward and Understanding of the Relationship Between the Quality and Cost of Hospital Care,* PhD Dissertation, University of Michigan, Ann Arbor, MI, 1989.
6. Garber, A.M., Fuchs, V.R., Silverman, J.F., "Case Mix, Costs, and Outcomes: Differences Between Faculty and Community Services in a University Hospital", *New England Journal of Medicine,* Vol. 310, No. 19, 1984.
7. Flood, A.B.W., Ewy, W., Scott, W.R. et al., "The Relationship Between Intensity and Duration of Medical Services and Outcomes for Hospitalized Patients", *Medical Care,* Vol, 17, No. 11, 1979.
8. Fleming, S.T., "The Relation Between Quality and Cost: Pure and Simple", *Inquiry,* Vol. 28, No. 2, 1991. See also Scott, R.W., Flood, A.B., "Cost and Quality of Hospital Care: A Review of the Literature", *Medical Care Review,* Vol. 41, No. 1, 1984; Fleming, S.T., "The Relationship Between Cost and Quality of Hospital Care", *Medical Care Review,* Vol. 47, No. 4, 1990. Roemer, M.I., Moustafa, A.T. and Hopkins, C.E., "Proposed Hospital Quality Index: Hospital Death Rates Adjusted for Case Severity", *Health Services Research,* Vol. 3, Summer 1968. Longest, B.B., "An Empirical Analysis of the Quality/Cost Relationship", *Hospital & Health Services Administration,* Vol. 23, No. 4, Fall 1978. Neuhauser, D., *The Relationship Between Administrative Activities and Hospital Performance,* Chicago Center for Health Administration Studies, Research Series No. 28, University of Chicago, Chicago, IL, 1971. Scott, W.R., Forrest, W.H. and Brown, B.W., "Hospital Structure and Postoperative Mortality and Morbidity", in Shortell, S.M. and Brown, M. (eds),

Organizational Research in Hospitals, Inquiry Books, Blue Cross Blue Shield Association, Chicago, IL, 1976.

9. Garvin, D.A., *Managing Quality*, Free Press, New York, 1988. Phillips, L.W. et al., "Product Quality, Cost Position and Business Performance: A Test of Some Key Hypotheses", *Journal of Marketing*, Vol. 47, No. 1983. Farris, P.W. and Reibstein, D.J., "How Prices, Ad Expenditures and Profits Are Linked", *Harvard Business Review*, Vol. 57, No. 6, 1979. Schoeffler, S., Buzzell, R.D. and Heany, D.F., "Impact of Strategic Planning on Profit Performance", *Harvard Business Review*, Vol. 52, No. 2, 1974.

10. Cleverly, W.O., Improving Financial Performance: A Study of 50 Hospitals", *Hospital and Health Services Administration*, Vol. 35, No. 2, 1990.

11. Harkey, J. and Vraciu, R., "Quality of Health Care and Financial Performance: Is There a Link?", *Health Care Management Review*, Vol. 17, No. 4, 1992. A follow-up inquiry by the author revealed that the study has not been repeated or updated in its original form. According to Elroy Schuler of that Organization, HealthTrust was acquired by Columbia/MCA on April 24 1995, and a new study has been undertaken concentrating on patient surveys, the specific results of which could not be revealed.

12. For an extensive review of these and related issues the reader is referred back to Chapters 2, 3 and 4 of this volume.

13. For an extensive discussion of these and related issues see Baumol, W.J., "On The Social Rate of Discount", *American Economic Review*, Vol. 58, 1968.

14. Bloomquist, G.C., "The Value of Human Life: An Empirical Perspective", *Economic Inquiry*, Vol. 19, 1981 (discusses the human capital approach). See also Linnerooth, J., "The Value of Human Life: A Review of the Models", *Economic Inquiry*, Vol. 17, 1979, and Berger, M.C. et al., "Valuing Changes in Health Risks: A Comparison in Alternative Measures", Vol. 53, 1987.

15. Goddeeris, J.H. and Bronken, T.P., "Benefit-Cost Analysis of Screening", *Medical Care*, Vol. 23, 1985.

16. Brook, R.H., "Appropriateness of Acute Medical Care for the Elderly: An Analysis of the Literature", *Health Policy*, Vol. 14, 1990.

17. Layel, J.R. et al., "Economic Impact of Preventive Medicine", *Preventive Medicine USA*, Prodict, New York, 1976.

9 Monitoring Healthcare Quality by Assurance

The healthcare process constitutes a complex interaction of various service components including inputs from the patient, one or more individual providers, healthcare institutions, and third-party payers and regulators. The perception of healthcare quality by each of these participants or participant groups may be quite different, depending on the perspective from which they see the process. Thus, a patient and his/her physician may see quality in a private or personal context, while private sector and public third-party payers and regulators see it more aggregately, typically from the perspective of some prevailing policy or even political objectives. Furthermore, the process needs to be examined and monitored in a dynamic context emanating from a frequently changing scientific base, medical standards, discoveries, and various practice patterns which utilize even established knowledge and standards with different efficiency as well as philosophy, at various stages of any given healthcare process within some structural setting aimed at a specific outcome. As a result, parties to the healthcare service delivery process have differing designs for, contributions to, and expectations from any quality monitoring system imposed on that process. Various questions may emanate from this labyrinth of concerned and interest groups. Should all care be monitored and at all times? If the answer is likely to be "no", then what aspects of care should be given priority, and what care-specific factors should contribute the decision of choice: volume, risk, patient attributes, or vulnerability to problems? And, how should the monitoring process be implemented: with what intensity, how close to the process of implementation without infringing on physician autonomy, all in consistency with prevailing policy and risk management and political goals?

The medical profession did not wait for society to remind it that some sort of monitoring process was in order, although it may have waited for social reminders to actually implement and particularly enforce those measures. The presence of professional responsibility to monitor care has been emphasized since 1918 by voluntary accreditation standards of hospitals requiring medical staff to regularly review and analyze clinical experience throughout the institution[1]. Attention to these issues was heightened by the entry of judicial and legislative sectors. The former by an increasing frequency of medical malpractice suits, while the latter with a barrage of regulatory measures at state and federal government levels. Nevertheless, many problems and issues remain in connection with the design and implementation of quality assurance programs which concern private interests as well as social welfare.

Quality Assurance Rudimentaries and Dilemmas

Although the topic of quality assurance has at a number of times been alluded to in this volume, they were glanced at within the context of other issues. Let us now examine some of the major dimensions of this monitoring process *per se*. Perhaps the best way to start a discussion of quality assurance is to warn that it is basically undefined, largely undelineated, and most attempts thus far to define and delineate it were plagued with all sorts of problems. Even in terminology, it may be questioned whether healthcare quality can be actually "ensured" or at best can only be protected. That is, if we have adequately defined what we are trying to protect, i.e. what is healthcare quality (these issues have been examined extensively in chapters 3-5). What is healthcare trying to achieve and at what acceptable cost? An acceptable answer would probably suggest something along the lines that healthcare should contribute to the patient's well-being at a socially acceptable cost. What level should the patient's well-being reach? Presumably, the higher is the attained level of well-being, the higher the quality of care may be, provided that the attained level of well-being is solely a function of the care provided. What if it is not, as it probably *is* not? Then, care quality may be identified in terms of the degree to which it contributes to, or increases, the probability that a desired outcome in the patient's health status is attained, or that a negative outcome for the patient is avoided or mitigated, subject to prevailing care standards at a community or national level. What is socially acceptable and unacceptable in terms of cost? An feasible answer may suggest that acceptability in this regard is both a relative and absolute concept: cost level should be viewed in terms of its proportion of gross domestic product, and how it compares with similar proportions for other national expenditure items. But, what should a desirable proportion be and how should it compare with other proportions? The answer is likely to be politically based and probably so implemented[2]. Notwithstanding these queries, some publicly sponsored quality assurance programs were and are implemented, although with not unexpectedly limited success. State medical boards have been exercising external control, but practice and sanction implementation were inconsistent among the states[3]. To strengthen state-based control efforts, the HCFA has for some time been ranking hospitals and physicians who service Medicare beneficiaries. For a while, largely unadjusted mortality rates were used to rank hospitals. Thus, factors such as patient population, case and procedure mix, were not used to adjust the outcome based on mortality. The effort turned out to be unwelcome in the healthcare community and in its original form it is now largely abandoned.[4].

Quality assurance programs often use process-specific terms and rely on definitions with their unique meaning for the efforts at hand. Thus, the term "norm" depicts statistical measures or standards for prevailing clinical practice. "Criteria" delineate proper clinical care in terms of frequently discussed structure, process and outcome dimensions; it entails explicit and implicit classifications, and so called descriptive referents (diagnosis, condition, treatment). "Standards" refer to some objective or quantitative statements regarding accepted or required treatments. "Flags" point to treatment areas that call for closer scrutiny. In addition to these, and perhaps a multitude of other lesser terms, some definitions often dominate quality assurance programs. Thus, in connection with the treatment *process*, efficacy, propriety, and caring are frequently assessed in terms of clinical trials, medical record reviews and patient surveys, respectively. Process itself is often assessed in terms of medical records and utilizations reviews. *Structure* normally, although not exclusively, refers to physician/patient bed ratios. *Outcome* considerations include mortality, intra-hospital infections and complications, health status, and post-care patient perceptions. Even the notion of quality itself can be seen in three different contexts: technical, optimal, and logical. "Technical quality" entails a comparison between actual and expected outcomes; "optimal quality" views outcome in the light of incurred costs; and, "logical quality" refers to the efficiency with which relevant information is utilized in the process[5]. Additional dimensions of quality assurance may cover items like access to care, the frequency and impact of medical malpractice suits, patient preferences, scheduling efficiency, length-of-stay, drug prescription patterns, and many more. In general, these terms, concepts and definitions, as well as their interpretations, vary widely among quality assurance programs and institutions. In addition, the terms quality "assurance" and quality "assessment" appear to have been used interchangeably in the literature although "assurance" has also been interpreted as a corrective action taken in response to some feedback ("assessment").

Inpatient Mortality and Care-Based Quality Assurance Models

A privately developed care monitoring system for Medicare patients suggested that hospital and diagnostic-specific (age and gender adjusted) mortality indicators can be generated, which would be subject to systematic and regular statistical analyses with inputs from hospital, patient, physician and third-party payer groups[6]. While theoretically feasible, the implementation of this plan would have been very costly, where costs would clearly need also to include the expenses incurred in connection with the repeated cost-benefit analyses to test the project's viability in different environments and at different times. Nevertheless, similar project proposals followed from HCFA. Thus, a 1986 model accounted for 59% of the variance in mortality and produced an expected death rate for each of some 5,500 hospitals surveys, utilizing variables such as age, gender, race, average length of stay, and the percentage that admissions represented of the most frequent DRGs. While the model was used, HCFA adjusted and refined it during each subsequent year, although during the initial years there was no adjustment for illness severity, and even in subsequent years factors such as primary patient diagnosis which has been shown to closely bear on mortality expectation, were not given adequate emphases. In 1987, an examination of deaths that occurred within 30 days of admission at these hospitals was added to the model. In 1988, techniques for medical record analyses were implemented in order to predict diagnosis-specific mortality. Similar improvements were implemented in subsequent years while the model remained in active use and application[7].

Private hospital-based mortality models attempted to separate out the frequency of preventable deaths from all mortality data. Thus, a study in the mid-1980s found a significant inverse relationship between inpatient mortality rate and the frequency of cardiac catherization in over 700 hospitals, when adjusting for case-mix. An expanded version of the same study a couple of years later looked at ten surgical procedures and similarly found a positive relationship between patient volume and outcome, that is, mortality varying inversely with procedure frequency[8]. Another study found that deaths in eleven hospitals exceeded predicted levels by over two standard deviations when deaths rates were adjusted for such factors as age, patient origin from a nursing home or from the ER, and DRG-based case mixes[9].

Diagnoses of strokes, bacterial pneumonia, myocardial infarction, and congestive heart failure for Medicare patients based on a 10% sample from a 1985 Medicare Provider Analysis Record file were found to account for some 31% of the Medicare 30-day mortality. Almost double the length of hospital stay and 25% higher inpatient mortality was found for these conditions in New York than in California, perhaps pointing to more effective quality assurance programs for Medicare beneficiaries in California than in New York[10]. Furthermore, there are some indications that cost-containment efforts accompanied by quality assurance programs tend to sustain quality at least at a constant level. Thus, a study of the Hospital Experimental Payments Program in Rochester New York during the early 1980s pointed to an increase in percapita healthcare costs some 50% lower than the national average accompanied by no significant changes in in-patient death-rates[11].

In addition to mortality-based studies, researchers also attempted to assess the effectiveness of quality assurance programs by way of so called "care appropriateness models" where care appropriateness may be viewed in terms of under or over-utilization (the medical necessity for and the correct process of care), and technically deficient service applications. Thus, a study of Medicare patients subjected to coronary-angiographies and carotid endarterectomies found inappropriate procedure applications in 17% and 32% of the cases, respectively, and counter-indications for these procedures in 9% and 32% of the cases, respectively[12]. In most instances, however, there is a blurred conceptual line between the appropriateness of service applications and the quality of care delivered because the former is often determined or profoundly influenced by the latter, and it is the latter that ultimately constitutes the target of most queries. In other words, service appropriateness may be difficult to separate out for examination, in spite of the fact that most quality assurance programs tend to target care processes rather than outcomes.

An attempt at systematically analyzing care appropriateness related issues was made at Boston University by way of a so called "appropriateness evaluation protocol" [AEP]. The system was designed to report on physician technical care as reflected by the medical records. AEP was to be applied to the medical charts of medical, surgical and gynecological patients by professional chart abstracters, regardless of diagnosis, in order to assess utilization rates[13]. However, the traditional elements of technical clinical care have at times been viewed as insufficient for implementing quality assurance and care quality control. The psychological input of the patient also became an important element of care quality control. Thus, factors such as patient attitudes, goals, expectations, health status and quality of life have come to be viewed as essential for quality assurance programs. Since these are rarely noted formally by the providers, some studies urged that they be routinely included patient charts[14].

Outcome Targeted Quality Assurance

Some researchers feel that quality assurance should improve the outcome of healthcare through better health, functional ability, well-being and patient satisfaction[15]. We noted that good care quality often suggests efficiency, equity, effectiveness, access, scientific and technical quality, among others. These entail structural and process dimensions not necessarily in causal relationship to outcome. Yet, quality assurance efforts have often utilized these structural and process dimensions with questionable implications for improved outcome. Furthermore, we noted earlier that outcome evaluations tend to be less than perfect. Patient-specific and environmental factors are not adequately accounted for. The process-outcome relationship is not always clear and at times is quite obscure. Case-mix variations in terms of severity and comorbidity are not or cannot always be taken into consideration. We elaborated on the various problems associated with the time dimensions involved in outcome measurements, i.e. the so called "optimal time window": at what time or stage of the recovery process can outcome, final outcome, be measured. In fact, other than with mortality, when can outcome be viewed as "final". Other problems such as patient-specific considerations and perceptions, cost-feasibility issues, adequate care standards, and patient volume are significant in assessing outcome pursuant to quality assurance[16].

Outcome targeted quality assurance may seek so called "efficacy" or, in the alternative, at the least so called "effectiveness". The former is normally perceived as the *ideal* application of optimal medical technology to some specific medical condition, while the latter is understood as the average or normal application of that technology[17]. The two differ in terms of the care environment, with the former viewed under ideal or even experimental circumstances, while the latter in more "real life" situations. Efficacy is best measured by well designed randomized clinical trials, when possible. If not, large databank-generated information may be utilized to estimate efficacy.

Patient satisfaction studies have also been used to assess outcome and the direction of quality assurance programs. These efforts are relatively new and have been questioned as to the aspects of care to which they may apply.

In general, they appeared to have yielded more reliable results with respect to the interpersonal aspects of the care than for the technical aspects. Nevertheless, and regardless of their reliability in terms of the technical aspects of care, patient feedbacks are considered essential for they normally govern patient (customer) behavior in a marketing sense. Whether they understand or appreciate the technical aspects of care, patients conduct their doctor search, disenrollment from prepaid care plans, compliance with physician advice, and other aspects of care that depends on them mainly on the basis of their perception of the care source[18].

All of these considerations point to a need to develop meaningful quality assurance goals in terms of some outcome considerations and targets. These targets need to be measured in terms of appropriate outcome related data. The quality and relevance of the data in turn clearly need to be assessed to see if it meets certain standards such as those established by the patient, the patient's family, the JCHO, HCFA, the state PRO, and other regulatory agencies. A method whereby quality assurance and related outcomes can be assessed is by seeing if patients treated in the same diagnostic categories experience similar outcomes. This would indicate care quality consistency as well as control over implemented care processes by QA professionals, but would require means of care process measurements, in other words relevant statistics. Quantifying care process and outcome is essential for quality assurance and relevant policy implementation. Relevant statistics allow the measurement and monitoring of care processes and resulting outcomes both while in progress and in terms of their final status. These statistics can be directly derived from the patient's experience with care. Thus, blood pressure, temperature, and pulse measurements are taken frequently and routinely. They are recorded on data-sheets and charts of various forms. Physicians also receive data from laboratories addressing the patient's health status at any stage of the care process. These data and related patient-specific information contribute to the provider's decisions regarding the care process elements to be implemented, as well as constitute inputs into the statistical datafile for the patient and in the aggregate for QA purposes.

Patient care standards and protocols have been developed and contrasted with patient specific data in order to ascertain consistency and deviations. These however may also be a source for problems in QA processes because while similarities might be striking, the treatment for the same illness but for two or more different people may call for different care inputs at some stage of the care process or another, the difference and deviation depending on the individuals involved. Identical illnesses for different patients may call for different care processes in order to generate identical outcomes, or identical care processes will generate different outcomes for different patients. Yet, there are clearly some patterns based on simple statistical principles. Thus, measurement data of the same nature when presented by way of a frequency distribution tend to gravitate towards the mean. If the data forms something like a normal curve then over two-thirds (68%) of the observations will be clustered right in the middle, 14% of the data will be in the next stage of both sides in the distribution, and only 4% of the data will be located at the high and low ends of the distribution. In other words, while variations in outcomes from the same care process do occur their range is in general predictable with specific probabilities, provided the variations are due to so called chance causes, i.e. those that are constantly present in the process and normally cannot be controlled or even detected. The other category of causes for variation, so called assignable causes, can be controlled and detected as they are not normally part of the process. Their presence, however, distorts the shape of the distribution (normal curve) and undermine the predictability of outcomes.

HCFA's Current and Planned Quality Assurance Efforts

Serious interest in monitoring healthcare quality intensified after World War II, particularly with the passage of Medicare in 1965 and subsequently with the establishment of the JCAHO which required that in order to be accredited a hospital must have an internal quality assurance program. The movement to monitor care quality, and in particular the recognition of the need to do so, gained further momentum in the mid-1980s when HHS began promoting the use of HMOs by Medicare beneficiaries, where HMOs were paid on a capitated basis, that is, all medical care was to be delivered to a beneficiary for a predetermined monthly payment per beneficiary. This was happening as interest in care quality, particularly as to care delivered by HMOs, was also increasing on the part of state regulators and large private purchasers or purchaser groups of healthcare services.

Care quality as perceived by HCFA typically includes the elements of appropriateness, technical excellence, accessibility, and acceptability. Appropriateness entails the right care at the right time. Technical excellence is present when care is delivered properly. Access indicates the ease with which needed care can be procured by the patient, and when the provided care is satisfactory from the patient's point of view acceptability prevails. As we noted in earlier chapters, these quality indicators are sought in the structure (institutional and resource environment, including physician and institutional credentials), process (the actual delivery of care) and outcome (the results for patients, however and whenever measured) of care.

There are two general approaches to quality assurance that were followed or are considered for implementation by HCFA. The traditional approach is basically an adversarial one between the provider and the reviewer whereby the former is scrutinized by the latter in a process designed to seek malfeasances. However, this process does not uncover those providers who do not actually malfease or who do not provide substandard care but function barely above required standards. In other words, the traditional approach does not differentiate between those services that are barely passable and those that provide excellent service. This apparent shortcoming is remedied by the so called "continuous quality improvement" approach to quality assurance which does not rely on specific past performances as much it attempts to improve present and future performance on the part of all providers regardless of the status of current performance. In addition, beside ascertaining structural dimensions such as credentialing, licensing and certification the private sector also takes into consideration outcome dimensions such as health status and patient perceptions.

At the present time HCFA has three broad measures to ascertain quality standards[19]. The first one established with Medicare in 1965, the *Medicare Provider Certification Program*, was aimed mainly at fee-for-service institutional providers such as hospitals, nursing homes, and home care facilities that need to meet a host of structural conditions, at least by way of rules and policies in place, in order to qualify for reimbursement. Individual providers' state licensing qualifies them for Medicare reimbursement. State agencies, under contract with HCFA, perform on-site surveys of institutional providers in order to ascertain that the conditions for accreditation have been met. A number of private third-party agencies' (such as JCAHO, some associations, societies, and commissions) accreditation is also acceptable by HCFA if the standards are at least as high as those of HCFA. Yet, there appear to be some doubts as how willing HCFA is to close down inadequate care facilities, except in extreme cases[20].

The second measure employed by HCFA to monitor quality standards relates to *HMO*s that serve Medicare beneficiaries. HCFA has typically had two types of contracts with HMOs: risk and cost. A risk contract entails a fixed amount per beneficiary paid to the HMO. This amount is normally based on the average Medicare cost for all beneficiaries in the particular

HMO's service area. Under a cost contract HMOs are paid a predetermined monthly sum per beneficiary based on a total estimated budget. To qualify for either type of contract, an HMO must meet the applicable standards of the Public Health Service Act and of the relevant Medicare statute. However, as with the Medicare Provider Certification Program discussed earlier, most of these standards are of a structural rather than outcome or even process nature, and, once again, questions have been raised as to the rigor and consistency of their enforcement[21].

While peer reviews, as tools for quality monitoring, will be examined at greater detail in the following chapter, it should be noted here that the Medicare Peer Review Organization Program does constitute an additional effort on HCFA's part to enforce some quality standards for Medicare beneficiaries, although mostly for fee-for-service surgical cases in hospital inpatient and ambulatory environments. The program appears to have two dimensions: process and to an extent outcome. Its process dimension focuses on reviewing patient charts, whereas its outcome related effort points to examining hospital-based adverse events [deaths, morbidity, infections, etc.], and early [within fifteen days after discharge] readmissions into hospitals. The PRO monitoring of care quality provided by risk HMOs dates back to a 1987 Congressional mandate. Beyond the HMO sector, HCFA's monitoring efforts are still largely restricted to hospital inpatient care, with minimum coverage of fee-for-service ambulatory care provided to Medicare beneficiaries beyond ambulatory surgical procedures. Some pilot projects covering these services are now under way monitoring the fee-for-service care of diabetics and other specific areas of care in ambulatory settings. In addition, there are some significant projects on the drawing board.

The 1995 GAO study refers to several major plans at HCFA designed to upgrade quality assurance programs. These plans appear to focus on three areas for improvement or implementation: continuous quality improvement, enhanced performance measures, and patient reaction surveys. Continuous quality improvement, that is the ongoing monitoring of service at any level of quality or performance, is seen as an improvement over traditional models of review which center on individual practitioner malfeasance in an atmosphere of adversity normally unwelcome by physicians. Under this type of review procedure reviewers work with the reviewed by way of cooperative projects designed to elevate all phases of patient care throughout the care process, thus where possible avoiding the unpleasantness of disciplinary situations.

The Foundation for Accountability (Facct) is a new organization being formed by HCFA in cooperation with a number of large corporate purchasers of healthcare services representing over 80 million subscribers. Its main functions will include the compilation and review of performance measure related methods and data regarding process and particularly outcome in the various types of healthplans involved. It may be that participation in this effort will obviate internal quality assurance programs or bring about major improvements in them. Finally, HCFA's Office of the Actuary which surveys about 12,000 Medicare beneficiaries treated in fee-for-service environments regarding various quality aspects of care such as access, attained health status, and other quality related consumer perceptions, plans to expand the scope of the survey to managed care environments. These plans and developments are significant for future developments in quality enforcement. The proportion of the US population in total which qualifies for Medicare benefits is increasing. The proportion of those that qualify will, due to the increased frequency of age-related maladies, also need to rely on Medicare supported care with increasing frequency and intensity. Thus, effective care quality control measures planned or implemented by HCFA will reverberate throughout much of patient populations.

Notes

1. Davis, L., *Fellowship of Surgeons: A History of the American College of Surgeons*, American College of Surgeon, Chicago, IL, 1973. Roberts, J.S. and Walczak, R.M., "Quality Assurance: The Evolution and Current Status of the Joint Commission on Accreditation of Hospitals' Quality Assurance Standards", *Quality Review Bulletin,* Vol. 10, 1984.
2. Quality assurance is not to be confused with quality assessment. The latter entails efforts typically aimed at measuring and monitoring the quality of medical care while the latter aims at safeguarding and improving care quality. See Office of Technology Assessment, US Congress, *The Quality of Medical Care: Information for Consumers*, Publication # OTA-H-386, US Government Printing Office, Washington, DC, 1988.
3. Vladeck, B.C., "Quality Assurance Through External Controls", *Inquiry,* Vol. 25, 1988.
4. Ginsburg, P.B., Hammons, G.T., "Competition and the Quality of Care: The Importance of Information", *Inquiry,* Vol. 25, 1988. See also Mosteller, F., "Assessing Quality of Institutional Care", *American Journal of Public Health,* Vol. 77, 1987.
5. Bliersbach, C.M., "Quality Assurance in Healthcare: Current Challenges and Future Directions", *QRB,* Vol. 14, 1988. Donabedian, A., "Quality Assessment and Assurance: Unity of Purpose, Diversity of Means", *Inquiry,* Vol. 25, 1988. Caper, P., "Defining Quality in Medical Care, *Health Affairs,* Vol. 7, 1988. Bennett, W.G., Delafield, J.P. et al., "Quality Assurance in Ambulatory Care", *Academy of Medicine,* Vol. 64 (Suppl 2), 1989. Fauman, M.A., "Quality Assurance Monitoring in Psychiatry", *American Journal of Psychiatry,* Vol. 146, 1989.

6.   Brook, R.H. and Lohr, K.N., "Monitoring Quality of Care in the Medicare Program: Two Proposed Systems", *JAMA*, Vol. 258, 1987.
7.   United States General Accounting Office, *Medicare: An Assessment of HCFA's 1988 Mortality Analyses*, GAO/PEMD-88-11BR, US Government Printing Office, Washington, DC, 1988. United States General Accounting Office, *Medicare: Improved Patient Outcome Analyses Could Enhance Quality Assessment*, GAO/PEMD-88-23, US Government Printing Office, Washington, DC, 1988.
8.   Luft, H.S. and Hunt, S.S., "Evaluating Individual Hospital Quality Through Outcome Statistics", *JAMA*, Vol. 255, 1986, and Hughes, R.G., Hunt, S.S. and Luft, H.S., "Effect of Surgeon Volume and Hospital Volume on Quality of Care in Hospitals", *Medical Care*, Vol. 15, 1987.
9.   Dubois, R. W., Brook, R.H., Rogers, W.H., "Adjusted Hospital Deathrates: A Potential Screen for the Quality of Medical Care", *AHPH*, Vol. 77, 1987.
10. Jencks, S.F., Williams, D.K., Kay, T.L., "Assessing Hospital Associated Deaths from Discharge Data: The Role of Length of Stay and Comorbidities", *JAMA*, Vol. 260, 1988.
11. Hartman, S.E., Mukamel, D.B., "How Might a Low-cost System Look? Lessons from the Rochester Experience", *Medical Care*, Vol. 27, 1989.
12. Lohr, K.N., Schroeder, S.A., "A Strategy for Quality Assurance in Medicare" [Special Report], *New England Journal of Medicine*, Vol. 322, 1990.
13. Restuccia, J.D., Kreger, B.E. et al., "Factors Affecting Appropriateness of Hospital Use in Massachusetts", *Healthcare Financing Review*, Vol. 8, 1986.
14. Emery, D.E. and Schneiderman, L.J., "Cost Effectiveness Analysis in Healthcare", *Hasting Center Report*, Vol. 19, 1989. See also, Bliersbach, C.M., "Quality Assurance in Healthcare: Current Challenges and Future Decisions", *QRB*, Vol. 14, 1988. Steffen, G.E., "Quality Medical Care: A Definition", *JAMA*, Vol. 260, 1988.
15. World Health Organization (WHO), Regional Office for Europe, *Quality Assurance of Health Services 38th Session*, Technical Discussions, Copenhagen, Sept. 1988.
16. Office of Technology Assessment (OTA), *The Quality of Medical Care Information for Consumers*, US Government Printing Office, Washington, DC, 1988.
17. Office of Technology Assessment (OTA), *Assessing the Efficacy and Safety of Medical Technology*, US Government Printing Office, Washington, DC, 1978.
18. See note #16.
19. Much of this section is based on USGAO, *Medicare: Enhancing Health Care Quality Assurance*, Testimony of Carlotta C. Joyner Before Subcommittee on Health, Committee on Ways and Means, Subcommittee on Health and Environment, Committee on Commerce, House of Representatives, July 27, 1995. GAO/T-HEHS-95-224.
20. United States General Accounting Office, *Health Care: Actions to Terminate Problem Hospitals from Medicare Are Inadequate*, GAO/HRD-91-54, Sept 1991. Also cited in #19.
21. See Chapter 6 of this volume for an elaborate discussion of HMO rendered healthcare quality. Also see: United States General Accounting Office, *Medicare: PRO Review Does Not Ensure Quality of Care Provided by Risk HMOs*, GAO/HRD-91-48, March 1991. See also *An Act to Amend Title XIII of the Public Health Service Act to Revise and Extend the Program for the Establishment and Expansion of Health Maintenance Organizations*, Public Law 94-460, October 8, 1976 [90 Stat 1945]. Amendments to Title XIII of the Public Health Service Act.

10 Monitoring Care Quality by Peer Review

Although they have been evolving institutionally and functionally, and developing at various rates for well over a century, hospitals in the US have undergone profound changes during the past two decades[1]. Most healthcare providing institutions of the 1960s and even 1970s barely resemble present-day complex corporate entities. In the past, the physician was the patient's sole agent and rarely anyone scrutinized the doctor's work. Basically, the hospital was a bystanding though accommodating entity with no control over the treatment, providing little more than physical facilities and environment under the physician's supervision and undisputed mandate.

Today, a hospital's functional scope and range of responsibilities would virtually be unrecognizable within the context of the past. Most relevant for our purpose, a hospital is now directly accountable for the quality of care provided within its domain. In fact, responsibility for care quality now needs to be met by both the treating physician and the accommodating hospital, with the latter being accountable for the quality of the care environment it supplies as well as the quality of the care provided by the physicians within its domain. The hospital may be viewed as the institutional umbrella under which care is delivered by those it engages or associates at all levels of the care production process, rendering it accountable for the care it delivers, while retaining the accountability of those individual providers who also participate in the care process.

There were several factors which facilitated the evolution of the current status quo. Consumers of healthcare service products have become increasingly informed and educated as to their own needs and desired standards of care that meet those needs. In fact, we noted earlier that consumers survey responses are increasingly relied upon as input components for quality assessment programs, although rarely published. Additionally, the traditional image of all physicians as infallible super-human beings of the highest character, scientific training, and competence has been significantly weakened indeed often formally and publicly questioned by proliferating media output within and outside the medical profession itself, and by various judicial and quasi-judicial proceedings. It had been estimated already several years ago that even then some 3%-5%, or about 20,000 of the practicing physicians in the US regularly malpractice. Furthermore, even the AMA estimated that some 10% of the practicing physicians could be placed in some sort of "impeded" or "impaired" category due to psychiatric disorders or substance abuse or dependence[2]. Institutionally isolated one-on-one physician-patient relationships, prevailing patient mentality and even uninformed naiveté, paternalistically self-serving, self-protecting and often institutionalized policies, rules and less formal but just as effective conduct standards generated and sustained fertile grounds for the perpetuation of this predicament. The sick individual who needed physician care often suffered directly in terms of his or her health status. Society which needed to carry the financial burden and the nonfinancial consequences of this state of affairs also suffered. Healthcare costs were spiraling. Quality was largely unmonitored. The problem became a social, political and an economic preoccupation for all of society. Negative externalities by way of increased medical malpractice insurance coverage costs and dimuned reputation as well as patient confidence impacted even the best and most qualified physician practitioners. Only the emergence of social and political power-groups, the proliferation of medical malpractice suits against hospitals and physicians, and the increasing imposition of competition on medical markets wherein a hospital's reputation could be attained or lost through the quality of care, prompted profound changes on the medical care scene.

The delivery of care within the hospital has been transformed. Instead of individual physicians, now teams care for the patient, albeit subject to the oversight of the patient's doctor. The team includes nurses, physician assistants, nurse anesthetists, respiratory and a variety of other therapists, a list that continues to grow as some functions which have traditionally been performed by the physician are increasingly transferred to allied healthcare personnel in order to reduce the cost care delivery, although subjecting the impact upon the quality of care to debates of ever increasing intensity. In managing the team, the physician must apply not only his or her technical skills in medicine but some talents in management and human relations.

Running the entire hospital is in the hands of two management hierarchies: hospital management and the medical staff management. The former includes the hospital's chief executive officer and his administrative staff overseen by the hospitals board of trustees and directors. The latter normally entails various committees such the executive committee of practitioners, a credentials committee, and a peer review committee. The hospital's attempt to maintain a qualified medical staff is normally implemented through two functional categories: *credentialing* and *peer reviews*. Both allow the hospital's management to at least attempt to control and monitor medical staff competence. By way of credentialing, a committee seeks data and information (initially on an application form that contains education and licensing related information as well as references) regarding the physician's technical competence and his or her ability to work with others in the relevant settings. Medical malpractice history, if present, often yields information as to the ability or diligence of the physicians to provide reasonable and standard care.

Peer review processes are similar to those of credentialing. They are, however, conducted continuously to monitor the pattern of care. Because the process and performance reviewed tends to be highly technical, the reviewers themselves are the direct colleagues of the physician, often within the same speciality, hence the process is relatively restricted and often closed. Thus, the care monitoring scene is that of a continuous reliance of medically non-technical hospital administrators upon the technical judgment of physicians and specialists.

The peer review process is inhibited by a number of difficulties. The formulation of opinions and reporting thereupon is often inhibited by fear of law suits to which a reviewer may be subjected from a reviewed but offended professional. These issues will be discussed at greater length in the next chapter. Another factor inhibiting peer reviews relates to the professional and financial interdependence among physicians within an organization: most are part of a direct or indirect patient referral network. This is compounded by the fact that members of a peer review committee typically do not get paid. Thus, participating in these committees incurs an opportunity cost in terms of time, and may also generate resentment on the part of and patient loss from fellow physicians who have been subjected to a negative review, whereas a positive review is unlikely to generate significant additionally referred patient flow since such review is typically expected as "normal" by the reviewed physician. Furthermore, physicians typically do not have much vested in the hospital's financial condition, so long as the latter remains solvent and the latter does not undermine the quality of care which the physician intends to deliver to his or her patient and implicate or more likely actually involve the physician in malpractice litigation. Lastly, physician members of peer review committees may hesitate to undermine personal friendships and relationships with reviewed physicians simply because of some impersonal attachments to the care quality of an unknown patient - that is, if the reviewer's ethical standards do not override these considerations.

Under these circumstances, the relationship between peer review results and hospital characteristics may prove to be important in assessing the nature and value of hospital-specific peer reviews. Thus, some recent studies aimed at scrutinizing the relationships between hospital characteristics and care quality as determined by peer reviews. One such study found that hospital mortality HCFA adjusted rates were higher in public as well as private but for-profit institutions than in private non-profit hospitals. In addition, mortality rates were found to vary inversely with hospital occupancy rates, payroll expenses per bed, the board certified proportion of physicians and specialists, the RN proportion in nursing care, the level and sophistication of applied technology, the size of the hospital in terms of bed-count, and membership in the Council of Teaching Hospitals. The problem with this study however was directly vested in the problems associated with HFCA's hospital-specific adjusted mortality rate figures. The latter is the difference between observed hospital-specific mortality and predictable or predicted mortality rates based on patient-specific billing data and charts. However, HCFA's mortality rate calculations aimed at inter-hospital general care quality measurements and comparisons, even if correct which in itself has been questioned, did not take into account differences among hospitals in terms of the severity of patient illnesses, hence the figures were biased against hospitals which admitted a larger number of severely ill or terminal patients and in favor of those that admitted none or fewer by the nature of their patient census and the relevant market[3].

More recently, another study also looked at the relationship between various hospital characteristics and the quality of care. Instead of relying on HCFA's mortality rate statistics, the authors base hospital quality measurements on patient medical record reviews by peer review organizations (PROs)[4]. The results of this study indicate that some hospital characteristics appear to correlate with better care, where "better care" is defined in terms of lower problem frequencies discerned by peer review organizations. Hospital characteristics that appear to vary directly with care quality include the technical training of the medical staff, level of diagnostic and therapeutic technology applied, occupancy rate, and payroll expense by bed - the latter presumably gauges at least the volume of care targeted at each patient.

Private and Public Sector Peer Reviews

A focus of peer reviews has typically been the attempted monitoring of hospital service propriety. Such reviews appear to be warranted by some studies which suggest that between 10% and 30% of hospital admissions and inpatient days are inconsistent with accepted medical standards in terms of propriety and patient need, generating excessive care costs and interfering with cost-containment efforts[5]. It was those cost-containment efforts which were initiated by third-party payers in response to employer and government sector clamoring for lower healthcare costs which prompted an examination of peer review as a means to the end. Hospital utilization reviews (URs) are viewed as an important category of monitoring devices in this regard, although their ultimate impact on healthcare costs is not entirely clear, and has yet to be consistently demonstrated. The stage for hospital utilization reviews was originally set several years ago by the US Government's Professional Standards Review Organization (PSROs) efforts aimed at reducing or at least monitoring Medicare patient care[6]. Once again, the evidence whether or not these efforts have in fact reduced utilization or that they contributed to significant healthcare cost reductions has been at best inconsistent. Some studies suggested that the government's program had at best a minimum impact on utilization, or no impact at all on hospital lengths of stay. Other researchers found that URs has reduced hospital stays by up to 15%, but these studies have lost some credibility to their critiques who claimed that they were technically inadequate due to not having controlled for the impact of important covariant factors[7]. These studies concentrated on URs as a means of inpatient hospital monitoring. Other scholars focused on another program: mandatory second-opinions regarding surgical procedures which were first implemented by Medicare in Massachusetts, and by a New York Taft-Hartley welfare fund. These found more encouraging results by way of approximately 60%-80% savings in most cases[8].

Two relatively recent studies have returned to URs, and attempted to examine the impact of that program on utilization intensity, and inpatient care expenditures[9]. We will discuss their findings, and then continue by looking at public sector efforts to control utilization. These studies utilized 1984, 1985 and 1986 claims data and appear to improve on earlier studies in various ways. While earlier studies looked at specific cases and compared utilization at various stages of a case and projected utilization based on that comparison, this study encompasses various geographical locations and utilized data from a large number of insured groups, while controlling for a large number of variables such as enrollee characteristics, healthcare market and various benefit plan attributes. Additionally, all inpatient and outpatient expenditures were studied allowing for a scrutiny of the effects of utilization review prompted switches from inpatient to outpatient care. The findings include conclusions to the effect that utilization review programs can lower hospital utilization as well as healthcare expenditures. Inpatient days and healthcare expenditure levels were found to have been reduced at least once by 11% and 6% respectively, although no significant changes in the dynamic rates of growth or reduction over time in these variables were discernible. In general, the cost-containment impact of utilization reviews in the private sector was found to be more modest than previously thought.

The evolution of modern care quality monitoring systems in the *public sector* spans over a period of almost half century, going back to the 1950s. Thus, the Foundations for Medical Care, a physician sponsored movement in California, goes back to the 1950s. Post-Medicare public sector care monitoring activities in addition to the Joint Commission on Accreditation of Hospitals ["Hospitals" recently replaced by "Health Care Organizations"] and the so called "Medicare's Conditions of Participation" in the program itself, include Experimental Care Review Organizations (EMCROs), Professional Standards Review Organizations (PSROs) and Quality Control Peer Review Organizations (PROs). The functions and impact of these organizations in inpatient and ambulatory settings will be examined in the rest of this section.

The first Medicare related concerted review process was implemented in 1970 and lasted for about five years. *Experimental Medical Care Review Organizations* (EMCROs) were voluntarily formed by physicians in order to assess care given to Medicare and Medicaid patients. The function of these organizations included a review of inpatient and ambulatory patient records, while their efforts were funded by the National Center for Health Services Research and Development. A review of this program at the state level suggested some positive impact in Medicaid ambulatory care brought about by economic sanctions and by various educational programs aimed at practitioners[10].

Even before the EMCROs folded, the Social Security Amendment of 1972 set up the so called *Professional Standards Review Organizations* (PSROs) aimed at physician and institutional performance within the Medicare program[11]. The thrust of care scrutiny focused on three general areas: (a) meeting community based and recognized care standards; (b) the presence of documented need for the service; and (c) efficiency subject to minimum quality constraints. The purpose was to contain public medical costs and overutilization frequently found with fee-for-service programs, and to monitor quality[11]. The organizations were made up of local voluntarily participating physicians, were not profit motivated, covered between 30-40 hospitals and about 3,000 physicians in close to 200 regions, and were financed partly by Medicare Trust Fund resources and partly by special appropriations from Congress.

PSROs monitored utilization by preadmission certification for elective procedures, post-admission certification for nonelective procedures, and closely observed lengths of stay. In addition, so called "profiling", that is a review of patient care after the fact for certain care episodes or for entire care processes, was implemented. These profiles could be constructed for a private physician, hospital, nursing home, a patient or for a group of patients within the same general care category such as a DRG. Profiling's main purpose was to identify instances where care was substantially below (or possibly above) established standards. Profiling was effectively supplemented by Medical Care Evaluation (MCE) studies which focused on existing problems of rather specific nature and instance. Finally, and subject to budget constraints, some PSROs engaged in broader quality monitoring activities involving ancillary services such as, laboratory work, radiology, long-term care institutions, nursing homes, and the like[12]. Attempts were also made at evaluating ambulatory services, procedures outside a hospital's environment, such as in physician's offices and at freestanding clinics. However, because ambulatory care was, and is, by its very nature much more dispersed than inpatient care involving more providers and provider cites, and because medical market conditions prevailing 15-20 years ago allowed physicians to be more successful in resisting reviews of their office records than they do now, and, finally, since the financial impact of ambulatory care on the medical scene (particularly before the implementation of the hospital prospective payment system) was much smaller in relation to inpatient care than it is now, PSROs have not been very effective nor very pervasive on the ambulatory scene.

Thus, while in some areas PSROs were effective, in others they were less so. Their net impact on the medical quality, cost and utilization scene may be hard to consistently assess. It has been speculated that PSROs may have contributed to quality improvement more than to cost containment, a relatively disappointing outcome in an era of predominant preoccupation with cost containment[13]. In general, the PSRO experiment pointed to various problems that can be encountered through any highly dispersed organization with inadequate management, and with situations where the conflicting targets of quality improvement and cost containment need simultaneously be attained.

The questionable performance of PSROs led Congress during the 1980s to seek alternative means of care/cost monitoring; enter the *Utilization and Quality Control Peer Review Organizations*, or, as we know them today, the PROs. Although the fundamental aims of the PRO program, as did the PSROs, centered mainly on three service dimensions: propriety, need, and quality, the timing for the emergence of the PROs made them more prominent within the entire Medicare system. The emergence of the PROs parallels the initial stages of the Prospective Payment System's Diagnostic Related Groups (DRG) method for paying hospitals which was formally implemented in October 1983. Thus, the new monitoring system had new fields to survey.

While there are several, the main piece of law that impacted upon the development of the PROs was the Tax Equity and Fiscal Responsibility Act [TEFRA] of 1982[14]. In general, it was Congress' intention to give PROs local orientation by requiring local physician participation, as well as access by speciality and third-party payers. No entity or individual subject to review could function as part of a PRO. Financing PROs is implemented through competitive bids which also include a proposed set of functions and responsibilities to be performed, often called "scope of work" [SOW]. Contracts have typically been awarded initially two and later for three years, they are renewable but can also be terminated by either the PRO or by the DHHS. The SOWs may change from one contract cycle to another or may remain relatively stable, depending upon prevailing political and policy trends. However, there is a core set of functional requirements which seem to cross contract and PRO boundaries and which include quality screening, admission and discharge reviews, DRG validation and scrutiny of invasive procedures, and a review of patient coverage as well as risk management systems. These functions are routinely performed on a random sample of 3% of Medicare patients, plus on many additional cases that arise due to specific issues that may come to the PRO's attention at any time.

Confirmed quality or utilization problems are generally classified into three categories, so called "severity levels", based on the potential or actual occurrence of adverse effects on the patient: the lowest level of severity entails some sort of medical mismanagement with no potential for adverse effect, followed by one where there is a potential for a significant adverse effect, and the severest level where medical mismanagement has caused a significant adverse effect for the patient. The subjective nature of these criteria, and a lack of consistent definition of "significant" leave much of the relevant scrutiny and assessment up to the judgment of the PROs involved. When problems are encountered, the responsibility for imposing sanctions rests with the DHHS, not with the PROs. The DHHS in turn has typically delegated authority to the Office of the Inspector General which acts with the benefit of recommendations from the PRO.

As did their PSRO predecessors, the PRO program has encountered serious problems. One of the main problems appears to be the high variation among PROs in terms of their quality control efforts and apparent effectiveness. Some of this variation has been explained in terms of the various calculation methods for quality failures that PROs employed. Another reason may rest with different patient and provider mixes that PROs encounter in their respective areas. Efforts are continuing to improve and standardize care quality and utilization monitoring practices[15]. It is likely that the PRO program will be altered or adjusted to constantly changing needs in the future but its fundamental structure will not change, such as happened to the PSROs. It should be noted that although the PROs have replaced the PSROs, the PROs have retained a number of the PSRO's characteristics. Their general aims and purposes were essentially the same: to ascertain that the services reimbursed by the government for the care of Medicare beneficiaries were needed, proper, and of quality consistent with accepted standards. At least in much of their history, both programs appeared to concentrate more on service utilization and cost control by peers at the local level for inpatient care than on the quality of care for the elderly. Both programs were inadequately funded with moneys constituting no more than about 1% of the total Medicare budget. They displayed variations in their review methods, criteria and findings. However, the programs also differed in several ways. The PSROs were funded through grants whereas the PROs through competitive contract bids. The PSROs were born in an era different from that of the PROs, were shorter lived, and their functions or performance were not impacted by the later emerging DRG hospital payment system. Finally, today's PROs benefit from better Medicare statistics and much more sophisticated computer and information systems.

Healthcare Monitoring in Preferred Provider Organizations

Earlier in the volume, we have examined various care monitoring processes and their impact on managed care environments. We will now look at similar issues and problems in a *preferred provider* setting [PPOs]. Like managed care organizations, PPOs emerged as an attempt to contain escalating health-care costs with the provision, not available in most managed care environments, that patients retain free choice among a selected group of providers. Lacking established or standardized guidelines for their formation, PPOs are more diverse than uniform in terms of their organizational form, manner of functioning, and background sponsorship. If there is any single feature that is common to all PPOs it is the arrangement through which patients have the financial incentive to utilize "preferred providers", i.e. hospitals and physicians who participate in the arrangements along with the financial incentives of another nature accruing to providers for participating in the same arrangement. The patient receives a discount for using the preferred provider while the participating providers' patient volume increases along with the efficiency of claim processing. While the structure of a PPO is generally determined by local market conditions, the arrangement normally includes a group of providers who contract to provide their service to a pre-selected group of patients at a discount albeit on a traditional fee-for-service basis. The key elements in a PPO arrangement are the group of preferred providers, contracted fee schedules, utilization review, efficient provider claim processing, a monetary incentive in some form of discount for the patients to use the preferred providers, and, what often makes PPOs more attractive to patients than HMOs, freedom of choice by patients among members of the selected group of providers at a discount, or outside the group at the undiscounted standard fee.

Costs are expected to be controlled by utilization review processes and by the financial incentive on the part of the patient to choose the discount physician who, in turn, and with a target income level, is likely to be more efficient than non-participating providers. Furthermore, in this system much of the financial risk of excessive utilization falls on the patient, not on the PPO or the provider.

While there may be other dimensions for PPO classification, the best from a structural point of view appears to be based on sponsorship. The *hospital* sponsored PPO category includes those that are hospital or hospital chain affiliated as well as those that are jointly sponsored by physicians and hospitals. *Physician* sponsored PPOs also include those that are sponsored by medical groups. Some are sponsored by *commercial insurers*, and other third party payers such as BlueCross and BlueShield plans. In addition *private investors* and dependent entities such as union trusts and HMOs may also sponsor PPOs. Having extensive experience with the business, the Blues appear to have sponsored most of the PPOs so far. It may also be noted that PPO enrollment does not appear to be significantly influenced by the type of sponsor involved[16].

The rapid development of PPOs have been enhanced by a variety of largely economic factors. The main impetus for PPO growth appears to have come from the transformation of medicine from science/art into business, a process that may be called the "monetization of medicine". Medicine monetization was mainly sparked by the increasing sophistication and purchasing power of corporate and other organized buyers of medical services, and, in particular, by an increasingly aggressive application of that sophistication and power in response to spiraling healthcare costs constituting perpetually increasing proportions of employers' total cost structures. In addition, patient volume and velocity for physicians and hospitals has been steadily declining. The given or shrinking patient pie needs to be sliced into an ever increasing number of smaller slices. Competition for the patient in the medical marketplace has become fierce, and is still increasing. So is the number of physicians, although not the number of traditional institutional providers, i.e. hospitals. Thus, there is also an "internal squeezing effect" experienced in medicine. Physicians need hospitals and hospital affiliations to train and practice. Yet, the increasing number of physicians are met by a decreasing number of hospitals with decreasing capacity, causing a scramble for hospital based positions such as residencies and fellowships, and even for basic staff affiliations in community settings. PPOs have proven to be an effective means for increasing sales volume and reducing excess capacity and the number of empty beds, although the extent to which they actually mitigated excess capacity in the medical sector is still uncertain.

As many other types of managed care organizations have proven themselves not to be, PPOs are no panacea either. In fact, there are several areas where PPOs may encounter or cause serious problems. These areas include legislative or regulatory, possible adverse impact on competition, malpractice accountability, and, perhaps most pertinently, in connection with peer review efforts to control costs. On the regulatory/legislative scene, PPOs suffer from what could be called a "regulatory conflict" because even within a given jurisdiction several PPOs may be sponsored by different types of entities subjected to different regulatory standards and provisions. Multi-state PPOs may be faced with a variety of regulations within each state, although this problem may not be more serious for PPOs than those encountered by other multi-state entities. A solution by way of uniform federal regulation of PPOs may not be a viable one as PPOs are often a product of sponsors of different type themselves state regulated, causing PPOs to be subjected to a "regulatory squeeze".

The nature of PPO operation may make them vulnerable to at least the appearance of competitive restraints. Because of the coordinated, albeit lower, pricing, price fixing may be of concern. Other concerns by way of monopolization, exclusive dealing, concerted market division may also become relevant both on the part of regulatory enforcers as well as excluded providers[17]. In addition to competitive restraints, the possibility of medical malpractice liability is also relevant for most PPOs as they constitute more of a financial reward for successful litigation than individual providers, notwithstanding the latters' likely separate insurance. Finally, utilization review outcomes regarding PPO affiliated providers, indeed the utilization review process itself, may have a counter-productive impact on the reviewed providers because of their likely or perceived insurgence on long-cherished physician autonomy.

PPO utilization review programs normally include several provider functions. Pre-admission reviews aimed at service need determination, service review for admitted patients, and length-of-stay clarification. They may also require second opinions for certain types of elective procedures, HMO-type of gatekeeping for service channeling, physician profiling as to credentials and performance, and recommend physician termination. The utilization review procedure itself may be implemented by the PPO, an independent third-party, or by a provider group engaged by the PPO from within or outside the PPO. The latter may generate a conflict of interest between patient volume and overutilization if census velocity is artificially inflated. This may particularly be the case with utilization review programs in hospital sponsored PPOs, leaving independent third-party utilization review programs as the most viable ones for objective implementation. We might add that objective utilization review programs are perhaps even more delicate than those for HMOs due to thus far less developed intra-PPO quality assurance efforts.

Quality assurance efforts within PPOs are relatively unresearched, and are probably underdeveloped. The reasons for this likely rest with two typical PPO priorities, namely to procure a preferred provider group and control costs by utilization review programs, which leaves internal quality assurance to a consideration of lower priority. In addition, PPOs typically engage the services of fewer providers than do HMOs, making meaningful performance comparisons, an important ingredient of quality assurance, more difficult.

Furthermore, the relatively new PPO's drive to gain or increase market share in their communities also appeared to relegate internal quality assurance to secondary importance, placing patient volume, cost, profitability, and market-share in the forefront of operation. This predicament will likely change as PPOs further proliferate, receive more attention as well as scrutiny from consumer groups, competitors and regulators at various levels.

Obstacles to Effective Peer-Review Processes

Medical peer review is recognized as essential to providing quality medical care. Yet, historically there has been a certain amount of reluctance on the part of physicians to participate in the process[18]. Assuming any political benefits and future positive fallout away, and negative ones are more likely when peer-reviews yield adverse results for the reviewed physician, there are few tangible incentives to partake in the process. While staff privileges at most hospitals presume peer-review participation *per se*, it does not ensure that the participation will be effective, conscientious, or even impartial. While hospitals have been held liable for the malfeasance of their incompetent or negligent staff-members or affiliated practitioners, there does not seem to be published evidence available to the effect that members of peer-review committees were sanctioned or were held liable for failing to censure or not recommend the exclusion of incompetent physicians. Yet, physicians may be motivated to participate in order to protect their patients, or to facilitate hospital accreditation where the latter in the private sector requires the performance of peer-review. Peer-reviews are standard requirements for Medicare[19]. In the same time, there are powerful disincentives for members of a peer-review committee to perform even up to expected standards. Censuring a physician may result in the loss of his/her hospital staff privileges, when the latter is normally viewed as a prerequisite for practicing medicine in any community in the first place. Thus, with economic damages and injury to professional reputation likely to be substantial, defamation suits were not uncommon. Patient referrals were lost. Other litigation involving discrimination and antitrust charges would often follow[20]. Furthermore, the healthcare environment has become much more conducive for charging antitrust violations. Competition for patients increased both in institutional care and private physician markets. Hospitals need physicians and vice versa. The choice for this association, however, is made mostly by hospitals rather than physicians. Some physicians are chosen or retained for privileges, others are excluded or terminated which they often see as grounds for complaint. Perhaps more importantly, good medicine no longer means good quality of care but rather good care quality along with cost-effective implementation of that care.

One solution to peer-review committee members' vulnerability to law suits would be to maintain the records and much of the proceedings of the committee as privileged and confidential. Indeed, securing anonymity for members of the committee. Some states have passed laws that secured this environment. However, typically they did not apply in cases brought in the federal courts[21]. The most important recent case that appears to govern in this context was decided by the US Supreme Court in 1990 involving issues regarding what was under state law privileged documents and proceedings in an academic peer-review process[22]. In this case, involving denial of tenure to an Asian female faculty member who complained to the EPOCH of discrimination based on race, sex and national origin, the Court essentially discarded the previously state recognized privilege for documents and proceedings in academic peer-review environments and ordered the involved university to release the relevant documents pursuant to the EEC's subpoena. The Court asserted that Congress did not intend to extend first amendment rights to the application of "academic freedom" principles in "confidential" peer-review proceedings and to related documents and materials. These privileges have traditionally been invoked by universities and hospitals to ensure a frank and uninhibited evaluation of the candidate's credentials. While that process is clearly important, the privilege also sheltered participation in, or various destructive forms of boycott, these evaluation processes by member(s) of the peer-review group which were motivated not by objective, frank and uninhibited intentions but rather by political, personal and prejudicial predisposition. Thus, in addition to the technicalities of the law, and the Court's interpretation of various rules as well as the Constitution, a trade-off also needs to be dealt with: a trade-off between the unquestionable benefits of protecting the participants in a truly objective, professional and uninhibited evaluation process, and the monumental damage and sorrow that a destructive, personally, politically and bigotry motivated process can generate for a candidate. These processes are inherently subjective. Medical care quality is subjective. Performance of academics in a university environment is subjective. In a peer-review based evaluation process, they are all subject to "judgments", professional and personal "judgments", academic judgments, medical judgments. So, if the evaluators need the protection of the law to exercise and implement their judgments, with potentially disastrous consequences for the candidate if those judgments are negative, why should the candidate, the victim, not be accorded the same protection by way of proper and complete legal discovery under oath which would allow reasonable persons to scrutinize the deliberations and the deliberators, judgments, credentials and competence relevant to the process, even emotional stability, displayed conduct and attitudes, and all of the documents as well as materials generated or relied upon in the peer-review process? If one side is protected, so should be the other side. That is perhaps the main lesson of this recent case, and although the drama was played out in an environment involving academic appointment, its pertinence to the medical scene can hardly be doubted.

Notwithstanding hospital-based medical peer-review processes, which as we noted have been in effect for many years, Congress still remained concerned by the protection of patients due to the softness of remedies which were at times applied. In particular, the migration of incompetent physicians from hospital-to-hospital and from one state to another, and a lack of adequate communication among hospitals and state regulatory agencies to prevent the resurfacing of these practitioners in their new environments, prompted Congress to consider additional remedies. The Health Care Quality Improvement Act (HCQIA) was enacted in 1986[23]. The Act implements a national reporting system for all significantly negative peer-review determinations and litigation outcomes. This reporting system was implemented in 1990 under the DHHS as the National Practitioner Databank[24]. In addition, in return for a limited immunity from liability of hospitals and participants that may arise from the outcome of medical peer-review proceedings, hospitals are compelled to report all significantly negative review proceeding outcomes to the Databank. The next chapter will examine in considerable detail the development and provisions of the HCQIA, and in particular, the role and functions of the National Practitioner Data Bank.

Notes

1. For a brief review of more distant past and recent hospital developments, see Seplaki, L., *Cost and Competition in American Medicine: Theory, Policy and Institutions,* University Press of America, Lanham, MD, 1994, Ch.12.
2. See Statement by Representative Wyden, 132 Congressional Records H9954, October 14, 1986. See also Waxman, "Sounding Board: Medical Malpractice and Quality of Care", *New England Journal of Medicine,* Vol. 316, 1987. AMA Council on Mental Health, "The Sick Physician", *JAMA,* Vol. 223, 1973. Shapiro, J.,

Pinsker, K. and Shaler, "The Mentally Ill Physician as Practitioner", *JAMA*, Vol. 2323, 1975.

3. Hartz, A.J., Krakauer, H. L., Kuhn, E.M. et al., "Hospital Characteristics and Mortality Rates", *New England Journal of Medicine*, Vol. 329, 1989. See also *HFCA Medicare Hospital Mortality Information*, Publication No. 00640. Washington, DC, 1988. Lorh, K.N., "Outcome Measurements: Concepts and Questions", *Inquiry*, Vol. 25, 1988. Blumberg, M.S., "Comments on HCFA Hospital Death Rate Statistical Outliers", *Health Service Research*, Vol. 21, 1987. Fottler M.D., Slovensky, D.J., Rogers, S.J., "Public Release of Hospital Specific Death Rates. Guidelines for Healthcare Executives", *Hospital and Health Services Administration*, Vol. 32, 1987. Rosen, H.M., Green, B.A., "The HCFA Excess Mortality Lists: A Methodological Critique", *Hospitals and Health Services Administration*", Vol. 2, 1987. Hsia, D.C., Krushat, W.M., Fagan, A.B. et al., "Accuracy of Diagnostic Coding for Medicare Patients Under the Prospective-Payment System", *New England Journal of Medicine*, Vol. 318, 1988. Flood, A.B., Scott, W.R, "Conceptual and Methodological Issues in Measuring the Quality of Care in Hospitals", *Hospital Structure and Performance*, John Hopkins University Press, Baltimore, MD, 1987.

4. Kuhn, E.M., Hartz. A.J. et al., "The Relationship of Hospital Characteristics and the Results of Peer Review in Six Large States", *Medical Care*, Vol. 29, 1991.

5. Chassin, M., Siu, A.L. et al., "Does Inappropriate Use Explain Geographic Variations in the Use of Healthcare Services?", *JAMA*, Vol. 258, 1987. Strumwasser, I., Paranjbe, N.V. et al., "Determining Nonacute Hospital Stays", *Business and Health*, February 1987. Restuccia, J.D., Gertman, P.M. et al., "The Appropriateness of Hospital Use", *Health Affairs*, Vol. 3, 1984. Gertman, P., Restuccia, J., "The Appropriateness Evaluation Protocol: A Technique for Assessing Unnecessary Days of Hospital Care", *Medical Care*, Vol.19, 1981. Siu, A.L., Sonneberg, F.A. et al., "Inappropriate Use of Hospitals in a Randomized Trial of Health Insurance Plans", *New England Journal of Medicine*, Vol. 315, 1986.

6. These programs will be examined in depth both as to their development and substance later in this chapter.

7. Dobson, A., Greer, J.G. et al., "PSROs: Their Current Status and Their Impact to Date", *Inquiry*, Vol. 15, 1978. Institute of Medicine, *Assessing Quality in Healthcare: An Evaluation"*, National Academy of Sciences, Washington, DC, 1976. Congressional Budget Office, *The Effects of PSROs on Healthcare Costs: Current Findings and Future Evaluations*, Government Printing Office, Washington, DC, 1979. This study was updated by the CBO as *The Impact of PSROs on Healthcare Costs: Update of the CBO's 1979 Evaluation*, USGPO, Washington, DC, 1981.

8. Ruchlin, H.S., Finkel, M.L. et al., "The Efficacy of Second-Opinion Consultation Programs: Cost-Benefit Perspective", *Medical Care*, Vol. 20, 1982. See also Martin, S.G., Schwartz, M. et al., "Impact of Mandatory Second-Opinion Program on Medicaid Surgery Rates", *Medical Care*, Vol. 20, 1982.

9. Feldstein, P.J., Wickizer, T.M. and Wheeler, J.R., "Private Cost Containment: The Effects of Utilization Review Programs on Healthcare Use and Expenditures", *New England Journal of Medicine*, Vol. 318, 1988. More recently, Wickizer, T.M., Wheeler, J.R.C. and Feldstein, P.J., "Does Utilization Review Reduce Unnecessary Hospital Care and Contain Costs?", *Medical Care*, Vol. 27, 1989.

10. Lohr, K.N., Brook, R.H. and Kaufman, M.A., "Quality of Care in the New Mexico Medicaid Program (1971-75): The Effect of the New Mexico Experimental Medical Care Review Organization on the Use of Antibiotics for Common Infectious Diseases", *Medical Care*, Vol. 18, 1980.

11. P.L. 92-603.
12. Kane, R.A., Kane, R.L. et al., *The PSRO and the Nursing Home*: Vol. 1, *An Assessment of PSRO Long-term Care Review*, R-2459/1-HCFA, The Rand Corporation, Santa Monica, CA, 1979.
13. Lohr, K.N., *Peer Review Organizations: Quality Assurance in Medicare*, The Rand Corporation, P-7125, Santa Monica, CA, 1985. See also HCFA, *Professional Standards Review Organization 1979 Program Evaluation*, Pub. No. 03041, DHHS, Baltimore, 1980, and General Accounting Office, *Problems With Evaluating Cost Effectiveness of Professional Standards Review Organizations*, HRD 79-52, Washington, DC, 1979.
14. See Peer Review Improvement Act, Title I, Subtitle C of TEFRA, Public Law 97-248, amending Part B of Title XI of the Social Security Act. Other relevant pieces of legislation included the Social Security Amendments Act of 1983, Public Law 98-21; the Deficit Reduction Act [DEFRA] of 1984, Public Law 98-369; the Consolidated Omnibus Budget Reconciliation Act [COBRA] of 1985, Public Law 99-272; the Omnibus Budget Reconciliation Acts of 1986 and 1987, Public Laws 99-509 and 100-203; and the Medicare Medicaid Patient Program Protection Act of 1987, Public Law 93-100. In addition, various regulations oversee the functioning of the PRO system, such as the Administrative Procedure Act [APA].
15. For a review of the various dimensions of the problems, refer to General Accounting Office [GAO], *Medicare Improving Quality of Care Assessment and Assurance*, PEMD-88-10, Washington, DC, 1988. See also, GAO *Medicare PROs Extreme Variation in Organizational Structure and Activities*, PEMD-89-7FS, Washington, DC, 1988. Office of Inspector General [OIG], Office of Analysis and Inspection, Department of Health and Human Services, *The Utilization and Quality Control Peer Review Organization (PRO) Program Quality Review Activities*, Washington, DC, 1988. Prospective Payment Assessment Commission, Medicare Prospective Payment and the American Healthcare System, Report to Congress, Washington, DC, 1989.
16. See Seplaki, L., *Cost and Competition in American Medicine: Theory Policy and Institutions*, University Press of America, Lanham, MD, 1994, Ch.14
17. We will take a careful look at the antitrust ramifications of healthcare quality issues in the following chapter.
18. Comment, "The Medical Review Committee Privilege: A Jurisdictional Survey", *North Carolina Law Review*, Vol. 67, 1988.
19. Comment, "Health Care Quality Improvement Act of 1986: A Proposal for Interpretation of Its Protection", *St. Mary's Law Journal*, Vol. 20, 1989.
20. Comment, "Patrick v. Burget: Has the Death Knell Sounded for State Action Immunity in Peer Review Antitrust Suits?", *University of Pittsburg Law Review*, Vol. 51, 1990. See also Jatte, "The Health Care Quality Improvement Act: Antitrust Liability in Peer Review", *Tort and Insurance Law Journal*, Vol. 24, 1989.
21. Comment, see note 18, at pp.182-87 and 191. See also Memorial Hospital v. Shadur 664 F.2d 1058 (7th Cir 1981); Robinson v. Magovern 83 F.R.D. 79 (W.D.Pa, 1979); and, Shafer v. Parkview Memorial Hospital 593 F.Supp.61 (N.D. Ind. 1984).
22. University of Pennsylvania v. Equal Employment Opportunity Commission 110 S.Ct. 577 (1990).
23. Public Law No. 99-660 Title IV, #402, 100 tat.3784; U.S.C.A. 11101-11152 (West Pamph. 1991).
24. 55 Fed. Reg. 31, 239 (1990) codified at 45 C.F.R. #60, 1991.

11 The Legal Environment for Healthcare Quality: The Healthcare Quality Improvement Act

This chapter will examine issues which are related to cost containment, care quality, and the compromise of care quality often to attain cost containment. These issues arose because of historical cost escalation, third-party payer concerns with those escalation, cost control techniques implemented by third-party payers, physician and in general provider reactions to those techniques, and the derivative controversy as to what constitutes needed or unneeded care. A technique designed to restrict the dispensation of services to those which are in some way or another considered needed is a system of rewards/penalties for under/over service dispensation. In essence, providers are motivated to limit their services to what they view as needed and the rewards are designed to at least partially if not entirely make up for what otherwise would be an income loss due to the service curtailment. The physician thus may not incur a significant direct or immediate income loss due to service curtailment. If the curtailment, however, causes harm to the patient, derivative costs and income losses by way of medical malpractice awards may occur either directly to the provider, or indirectly to the provider by way of increased malpractice premiums charged by the insurance carrier, or both These pecuniary damages need to be considered in addition to indirect non-pecuniary ones from the litigation and particularly from its outcome, such as negative reputation and marketing fallouts, and entry into the National Practitioners Data Bank.

An issue core to the above is the determination of what is or should be considered "needed" and "unneeded" care. These notions are inherently relative to some standard(s) of care. Thus, the key questions: what should the standard of care be, how should it be defined, and measured? Standard of care defines and demarcates needed care from unneeded care. If unneeded care is provided it may not do any good, and may even be harmful if risks are involved, as they often are; if it is not provided unnecessary expenditures are avoided and costs are contained to that extent. If needed care is not provided the results may be serious for the patient, and although direct costs are contained to the extent of not providing the care, indirect or what may be labeled as "derivative costs" could be enormous if the patient sustains injury due to the omission. A category of these *derivative costs* is determined by way of malpractice litigation in the courts, where the latter are often called upon to delineate standards of care relevant to the case, a matter which will be discussed shortly. Another category of *derivative cost* relates to the economic wastage in the workplace (missed workdays, reduced output, and profits, etc.) and throughout the economy which needed care omissions cause by way of patient injury. A third category of *derivative costs* may be of a non-pecuniary nature, such as physical and emotional pain and suffering on the part of the injured patient, a category which may also cause pain and suffering to juries when they are called upon to quantify it in a medical malpractice suit. However, the *standard of care*, its definition and delineation remains the core concept in the entire process.

Yet, the *standard of care* can be an elusive concept. First of all, is it to be viewed as a minimum level of care that a specific patient with a specific ailment needs, or is it an average level of care which the same patient needs for the same ailment, or is it some optimum level of care for the same patient with the same ailment? Is it to change when the patient changes, or when the ailment to be treated changes? Last, but certainly not least, whatever the answers are to these questions, how do those answers change over time, given the fact that the art and science of medicine are constantly evolving and constitute a dynamic process over time. The courts have attempted to deal with these issues, i.e. establish standards of care, on a case-by-case basis as they were litigated. In general, it was found that the courts have been patient oriented, that is, gave the benefit of the doubt to the patient when a service was withheld often declaring the omitted service as needed[1].

These court decisions apparently reflect prevailing social conscience, but concern themselves very little, if at all, with principles of cost-containment *per se*. In that regard they are contradictory, for the medical cost-containment efforts themselves have been presented more as social and often political issues than issues reflecting private interest such as corporate bottom-lines. This is so notwithstanding the fact that much of the cost-containment efforts have lately been provoked and propagated more by corporate buyers of healthcare services than by social groups. Furthermore, patient orientation of the courts may actually be viewed as antisocial if large plaintiff's verdicts may have added to healthcare costs through increased malpractice premiums passed on to the patients, provided that passage is permitted by market and demand elasticity conditions.

Whether or not the outcome of a medical malpractice litigation, whatever that outcome may be, and the proceedings that lead to that outcome, should be viewed as reflections on some sort of established healthcare standards is questionable. It is tenuous even within the context of the specific case litigated, and may certainly not be applicable to other patient/care environments even if similar in some regards. The reasons for this is the myriad of nonmedical factors that interact during the litigation and throughout the trial. First of all, if the case settles the result is even less indicative of what care standards may apply in the case than if the case proceeds through trial and a verdict. The settlement outcome may be the result of many factors totally unrelated to the nature or standard of care applied. The relatively low amount of settlement may emanate simply from the attorney(s) proclivity to settle rather try a case. In some instances a plaintiff's attorney may find it financially expedient to settle for some amount less than what may be expected pursuant to a trial by way of a verdict if the mathematical expectation of the latter is lower than the settled amount. In other words, even a skilled, experienced, and completely ethical plaintiff's counsel would recommend acceptance of defense's settlement offer (S) if that offer exceeds or at least equals some expected verdict (V) times a reasonable probability (p) for that verdict being reached by a jury; that is, a settlement is called for if $S = pV$, or $S > pV$. This may be modified by allowing for litigation expenses (e) for the plaintiff, plus attorney's fees which is a constant proportion (f) in most cases the absolute value of which increases with the amount of S. Thus, this may be restated as a settlement acceptable from the claimant's point of view if $S - e = $ or $> pV$, or ideally $S - e - fS = $ or $> pV$. While S is known when an acceptable settlement offer is made, p is not. In fact, p may be difficult to determine even under what may appear to be the most predictable outcome circumstances. Many cases have gone to juries with the plaintiff's full expectation of a verdict along with some visions of an amount for the verdict, only to find that juries have come back either with defense verdicts, or with plaintiff's verdicts far lower than expected[2].

Since in cases of settlement, if the settlement occurs before key stages of the trial, there is no opportunity to enunciate and elaborate on standards of care by the two sides, the issues of care standard do not receive attention adequate for establishing those standards, even if the court was to establish that standard. Thus, whether or not the amount of settlement is indicative of the care standard breached even in that particular case is highly questionable. However, the settlement is likely to be the result of several other factors: relative attorney skills; differing standards and levels of attorney motivations. It is conceivable that some attorneys may accept cases for the single purpose of settling them, that is, never themselves intending to try the case, even if the value of **pV** is obviously high. The goal, the only goal, right from the stage of filing the complaint is to settle. In situations such as that, the amount of **S**, if reached, will likely be much lower than what **pV** would be, losing considerable portion of a recovery for the client, and a fraction of that by way of the attorney's fees. However, the loss of a fee-proportion is readily accepted by the attorney if the additional amount work and perhaps skill requirements for the case to be tried would be viewed by him/her unacceptable or insurmountable. Thus, once again, the settlement amount, **S**, means virtually nothing in terms of its possible role as a measure of deviations from accepted standards.

Even in cases where the attorney accepting the claim fully intends to pursue it and if necessary try it, the validity of a settlement amount as a yardstick of deviation from care standard is questionable. Once again, differences in relative attorney skills and reputation hence differing perceptions of a real threat by the opposing side, difficulties in discovery of relevant or correct information, differences in the skills and preparation of experts utilized by either or both sides, and other matters relating to competence, preparation, attitudes, case-loads, and so forth, all will impact upon the amount of settlement, but none of which directly bear upon the degree to which *standards of care* may have been compromised in the case at hand.

If the case is tried, and the jury returns a verdict, whether for the plaintiff or the defense, once again whoever gets the verdict does not necessarily indicate whether or not *care standards* were compromised. A defense verdict does not necessarily indicate that there was no infringement on some recognized community-based care standard any more than a plaintiff's verdict would indicate that there was. The list of reasons for this anomaly includes those items that I mentioned in the previous paragraph. However, in addition, we are now also faced with relative attorney skills in the courtroom, and they do indeed vary rather greatly, as well as juror predisposition, possible biases, cultural and socioeconomic backgrounds, as well as outright emotional factors. A dramatic and passionate presentation of the case by an attorney during trial followed by an equally dramatic and passionate closing argument to the jury could generate a substantial verdict amount factor, positive or negative, even if the jury comes back for the plaintiff. Once again, the amount of the ultimate verdict is much less likely to represent the extent to which *care standards* were actually violated than the myriad variety of perceptions that were designed and intentional generated for jury consumption during the trial by all of the actors and actresses with their many different roles in the court room drama. In other words, the outcome of medical malpractice litigation will unlikely generate any reliable yardsticks for measuring departures from care standards even in the latter stages of discovery and litigation, and certainly not in the earlier stages.

The difficulty of assessing care standards, and the extent of departures form those standards, however, becomes even more complex. Even if in any one case the court were able to generate reliable data for measuring deviations from care standards, each such case is likely to be vastly different from the next one. Ailments and patients vary from case to case, physician practice patterns differ, and various other differences and changes may make it impossible to translate court proceedings into some sort of yardstick for measuring deviations from care standards. Indeed, these standards may vary for the same ailment but from patient to patient, from one geographical location to another, from one time to another, and from one general or specific clinical situation to another. Patients and applicable medical treatments are far too diverse for the courts to generate some sort of universally acceptable set of standards. So, the criteria are reduced to mere "good medical practice" as seen customary and usual for the relevant communities[3]. This seems to be the case when the issue is whether or not a specific care service item should have been provided to the patient but was not, or when the controversy centers on whether or not that or another specific care service item has been performed properly.

Notwithstanding these problems, increasing exposure of both individual and institutional providers to medical liabilities in the courts forces the issue of dealing with some sort of norm relative to which a malfeasance of some sort can be established. Furthermore, it is really not up to the court to establish standards for medical care. Standards of acceptable care evolve through the interaction of members of the medical profession via scholarly journals, meetings, seminars and other scientific forums. In this manner, the process of establishing standards at any level is a dynamic one, and it is one that changes with time. Each time standards are set or changed, they are implemented for each disease treatment by way of practice protocols, or, so called practice parameters. These parameters are often developed and disseminated by speciality societies and academies, and by the National Institutes of Health[4]. Thus, it is up to the medical profession itself to establish standards, and, at least theoretically, leaving only the *enforcement* of those standards to the courts, even if the financial awards do not in fact measure the extent of deviations from those standards, as discussed earlier. The court will in most cases simply receive expert testimony from a physician as to what in his/her professional opinion the accepted standards are and how those standards apply, if they do, to the case at hand. In addition, even if the standards are met, they do not necessarily suggest that the care provided was in fact effective. Defense medical experts normally testify not to the effectiveness of the care complained of but rather that the care rendered was in conformance to some sort of pattern of medical practice which has been viewed as standard [accepted and customary] for the community. Furthermore, care standard, even if offered by the profession and accepted in some fashion by the courts, does not necessarily imply a *high quality* of care. Indeed, a standard that was accepted in a case cited no more than that possessed by "... minimally competent physicians in the same speciality..."; another case suggested a standard for a defendant provider in terms of the "average practitioner in the class to which he or she belongs"[5]. Let us now take a look at how society reacts when care standards, whatever they are in specific cases and under specific circumstances, are not met.

The Health Care Quality Improvement Act: The Background

Healthcare has long been a major national expenditure item in the US. It has also preoccupied us socially and politically for several decades. Having had healthcare in our social and political focus for so long, we would expect American medicine to be uniformly superior in quality, responsible to its consumers, and conscious of its role in and of its obligations to society. However, while much of medicine in the US may very well be the best in the world, there are and have always been causes for concern and sources of problems. There are weak spots in the delivery of healthcare in this country. These weak spots constituted at least part of the rationale for the passage of the Health Care Quality Improvement Act [HCQIA][6]. Let us briefly review some of the shortcomings in a system that prompted the design of legislative remedies.

Issues that precipitated legislative proposals with respect to healthcare delivery were initially mostly perceived and later actual medical malpractice crises. In fact, there appear to have been at least two relatively distinguishable waves of medical malpractice crises in recent decades. During the mid-1970s, the perception of a medical malpractice crises was predicated upon what was then seen as an explosion of medical malpractice litigation. Insurance rates increased by several hundred percent in one year, and in some states coverage has been restricted or outright withdrawn. Although there appeared to be no significant empirical evidence to support this crisis, many state legislatures enacted laws restricting the right of plaintiffs to sustain significant malpractice claims[7]. Nevertheless, the panic generated relatively stable insurance rate structures for the next decade. The second perhaps more substantive crisis seems to have erupted during the mid-1980s, when medical malpractice insurance costs to physicians have doubled from $2.5 billion to about $5 billion[8]. The blame was placed once again on extensive medical malpractice litigation, once again prompting states to further curb the claimants' rights to recover by way of additional "tort reforms"[9]. However, by this time countervailing voices have began to emerge directing attention away from tort actions as the source of the crisis into the direction of *insurance pricing* practices, and concerns for *physician competence* and diligence.

The main concern in connection with insurance pricing was predicated upon the fact that only a small fraction, something like 10%, of all the medical malpractice incidents, and one in seven of the major ones, actually resulted in claims, and then among those that were filed only about 4% actually received compensation[10]. In addition, the insurance industry, as do other industries, experience business cycles which affect their costs and earnings but may not at all be related to the filings of tort claims[11]. Finally, the increase in medical malpractice claims, and in the size of the awards, that was experienced during the late 1970s and the first half of the 1980s [which, incidentally, leveled off in subsequent years] and which was often referenced by insurance sources as excessive, was found by other industry professionals and experts as normal, consistent with cycles within the insurance industry, and, indeed, consistent with the trends in the various sectors of the medical industry itself[12]. Thus, increases in medical malpractice premiums were attributed to so-called "over-reserving" efforts by the insurance industry[13].

While alarming, the large number of incidents by way of medical negligence does not necessarily mean that physicians are incompetent. Medicine is by and large a high risk business, with often narrow margins for error, and serious consequences ensuing from errors. Thus, any physician, regardless of his/her level of competence, may encounter medical malpractice suits. Nevertheless, many indications of the presence of incompetent and unethical physicians have been asserted. Among them it has been alleged that some 5-10 of the physicians are incompetent. Some 15% of physicians become impaired through substance abuse at one time or another during their career[14]. Furthermore, it has been alleged that too few of the physicians who malfease were seriously disciplined. In most cases, the proceedings were kept quiet by way of a deal whereby the physician quietly surrendered his/her license in return for avoiding formal proceedings or even recording of the violation. The violator simply moved on to a different hospital or to another state to resume practice again, and likely commit the same violation[15].

A source of the problem rests with the limited capacity of state *licensing boards*. The licensing of doctors dates back to 1760 in the US. Every state engages in the process with various or limited degrees of effectiveness or adequacy. By and large, state licensing boards have been viewed ineffective in weeding out incompetent physicians[16]. Disciplinary actions of a serious nature that have been taken seem to center on areas of medical endeavor where malfeasance is relatively easy to prove and often are obvious, such as erroneous prescription writing, and alcohol abuse. Charges of a more complex nature such as incompetence are rarely adjudicated[17]. The reasons for this relative impotence of licensing boards seem to be related to limited budgets, the reluctance of board members to judge their peers or possibly friends, lack of adequate information to effectively pursue the matters, and finally although not conclusively the preoccupation of some licensing boards with protecting physicians against competition from non-physicians.

Medical malpractice litigation, to whatever extent experienced during the past twenty or so years, did not seem to ensure uniform healthcare quality either. One would hope that the threat of law suits, the financial and reputation exposure that it could bring, and possible other sanctions that could ensue from an adverse outcome, might deter the practice of substandard medicine. However, that system is not very comforting either. Even if a defendant physician loses, the financial sanctions imposed by the court [frequently excepting punitive damages] are borne by some insurance carrier or carriers which will likely set premiums more on the type of a physician's practice than on his/her track record. Furthermore, even in extreme cases of malfeasance, courts rarely had the authority or displayed proclivity to remove a practitioner from the medical scene. In addition, there are no indications that state licensing boards collect or in a disciplinary context utilize outcome data from medical malpractice litigation.

Another important component of the background scene for the enactment of the HCQIA relates to inadequacies in the *peer-review* process. As we noted earlier, the process which involved peer monitoring of physician performance is largely hospital-based and is mandatory whenever Medicare reimbursements are involved. The fact that the process is hospital based is essential in that the subjects of the evaluation work within the same environment and often in association with those physicians who have the expertise and the experience to observe and to conduct the evaluation continuously. However, peer-evaluation as a process designed to monitor and safeguard quality has demonstrated major shortcomings. Peers hesitate to judge peers, particularly when the outcome for the colleague's career may be serious, such as restricting or withdrawing the license to practice. Furthermore, there are no significant positive financial rewards for serving on peer-review committees, while there may be significant negative ones if past friendships or associations are lost impacting on the evaluators' future social or professional contacts. For some years, there has also been the threat of litigation involving defamation, denial of due process, and malicious interference with contractual or business relations[18]. To protect the evaluators, states enacted laws designed to provide immunity, although not insurance, in certain cases[19]. To deflect these laws, physicians started filing federal antitrust suits which allowed them access to otherwise confidential peer-review records, and which accorded them treble damages in winning cases[20]. Notwithstanding these problems, peer-reviews are still heavily relied upon and play an important role even within the implementation of the HCQIA, although the role of peer-reviews has been significantly supplemented by the establishment of a databank containing information regarding disciplinary actions against physicians.

The Health Care Quality Improvement Act: Legislative Developments

The legislative development of the HCQIA may be traced through the passage of three House of Representatives (HR) bills: 4390, 5110, 5540, with one Senate bill S.1744 culminating the process. HR 4390 was introduced by Congressman Wyden on March 12, 1986 with the hope that it would reduce medical malpractice in the US by formally subjecting negligence and incompetence to disciplinary actions[21]. The passage of the legislation appeared to have been accelerated by an antitrust suit of members of a disciplinary committee by a disciplined physician[22]. Dr Patrick's clinic privileges were terminated by members of a disciplinary committee. He countered by suing members of the committee, essentially claiming an antitrust conspiracy against him under the Sherman Act. Patrick won over $2 million [including a punitive elements by trebling] in damages at Federal District Court. The Ninth Circuit Court of Appeals reversed on the theory that the committee acted on behalf of the state, the process was state mandated, thus enjoyed state action immunity under the antitrust laws. The US Supreme Court reversed, finding that it was the hospital, instead of the state, that made the final decision regarding suspension of Dr Patrick's privileges; in fact, the state did not even have the power to review or reverse on merits the committee's decision, except on procedural grounds[23]. When introducing the bill, Congressman Wyden asserted that

> "The present system can penalize those doctors who blow the whistle on a colleague they believe is malpracticing. In Astoria, OR. where the physicians of a clinic reviewed another doctor's technical competence, the doctor sued them. ... Regardless of the guilt or innocence of the Astoria doctor, cases like this demonstrate that if this country wants physicians to come forward and prevent truly bad doctors from hurting people, there must be legal protection for them from the possibility of multimillion dollar litigation, years in court and financial ruin[24]."

HR.4390 provided legal immunity for physician participants of a peer-review. In addition, it set up a national clearing house for the collection and proper dissemination of adverse information on physicians. The immunity of peer-reviewers under federal law is predicated upon state certification that the review process took place in "good-faith", due process was accorded to the disciplined physician, all pertinent facts were obtained or that reasonable efforts were made to obtain those facts. The processes were assumed to be in good faith, unless "clear and convincing evidence" could be produced to the contrary - a difficult task. The national database regarding physicians was initially seen to collect data on malpractice related payments [judgments or settlements], and on sanctions imposed by state medical licensing agencies[25]. State actions were also to be reported to the USDHHS which was not to grant Medicare participation to hospitals unless the latter requested this type of information from HHS. In later stages of the Act's development, this requirement was replaced by an assumption that a potential Medicare participant hospital had knowledge of the physician database's relevant content. Note that disciplinary actions brought by hospital-based peer-review groups, perhaps the most frequent source for physician disciplinary actions, were not required to be reported by this first version of the Act.

HR.5110 contained important revisions of HR.4390[26]. State review committees were removed, which essentially gave the courts the primary responsibility for overseeing hospital-based peer review decisions. Immunity was extended to grievant lawsuits in both state and federal courts, provided that disciplinary actions against physicians were reported by peer-review groups to the USDHHS. However, HR.5110 did not make it any easier for the grievant to establish that disciplinary actions were not the result of pro-ceedings conducted in "good faith". It did impose the obligation on Medicare affiliated hospitals to procure HHS databased information on physicians considered for staff privileges.

Objections from federal antitrust enforcement agencies appear to have been a major force behind the decision to revise HR.5110, and to replace it with *HR.5540*[27]. While the bill revised the previous one in a number of areas, it appeared mainly to focus on issues related to immunity. Import-antly, the bill made it clear that peer-review processes are not immune from challenges by federal antitrust enforcement agencies, i.e. the Federal Trade Commission or the US Department of Justice's Antitrust Division. In addi-tion, the bill prevents disciplined physicians from recovering provided the peer-review committee met the designated immunity standards. Once again, federal enforcement agencies can seek penalties under the antitrust laws. The question-begging "good-faith" standard for immunity of HR.5110 was replaced by a so-called "reasonable belief" standard. The latter mandated that there be reasonable belief that the committee's action is in "furtherance of quality health care", and that such action was taken after "reasonable efforts to obtain the facts of the matter" and "after due process to the physi-cian involved"[28]. To further guard against anticompetitive abuses, the bill precluded immunity in actions aimed at issues other than those involving the physician's professional conduct or competence. For instance, issues preoc-cupying a peer-review committee such as competitive, promotion, or market-ing efforts undertaken by physicians and considered unprofessional by mem-bers of the peer-review committee could not be dealt with under the bill's immunity standards, and members of the committee could not be shielded against antitrust or other actions that the disciplined physician may bring[29]. After some further amendments, the bill was passed by the House, approved by the Senate as part of an omnibus bill S.1744, and signed into law by President Reagan[30].

National Practitioner Databank (NPDB)[31]

NPDB collects mainly negative information regarding physicians and disseminates that information to entities such as HMOs, hospitals, which retain the services of physicians, or to other organizations such as medical licensing boards, that have the responsibility to evaluate or credential physicians. As indicated earlier, reporting peer-review outcomes to the NPDB is a prerequisite for peer-review committee members having immunity against reprisals by the disciplined physicians. Such immunity, in turn, enables qualified peer-review committee members to function in their role as evaluators without being inhibited by the fear of reprisals from the disciplined physician, subject to the constrains imposed by the HCQIA upon the evaluation process, as we outlined earlier. The objective of the NPDB is to provide a centralized source of information on physicians in order to restrict the future options of medical malfeasers after the fact, which options would otherwise allow them to repeat their malpractice to the detriment of additional patients in the same or different parts of the country.

The statute mandates that report should be made to the databank whenever a *payment* is made on behalf of a practitioner in response to a claim of malpractice against him or her. Allowance is made for the possibility that some payments may have been made in cases where the claims had no merit in the first place: "A payment in settlement of a medical malpractice action or claim shall not be construed as creating a presumption that medical malpractice has occurred"[32]. Nevertheless, payments of all sort in response to claims are red-flags, and even if a claim is frivolous the consequent payment will have a negative connotation for the practitioner. Ironically, if a physician settled a claim by way of some arrangement which did not involve "payment", such as forgiving past patient bills or a commitment to render services to the patient at no cost for a specific time period, no reflection of the episode would appear in the NPDB. In reality, while it is possible to avoid "payment" by simply forgiving past patient bills, it is not likely that a claim would be settled by a commitment of future services by a practitioner where the claim arose from the inadequate competence of the same practitioner in the first place. Thus, while the rules may be wobbly in this regard, the consequences are not likely to be serious. An additional problem in this regard relates to the Act's specifying that payments made on behalf of a corporation instead of that of an individual practitioner are not reportable to NPDB. A publication issued subsequent to the Act, presumably to clarify some of the Act's provisions indicates, however, that if the payment is made on behalf of a one-person professional corporation such payment must be reported[33].

Another function of the NPDB is to receive information from state licensing boards as to restrictions or revocations (but not initial denial) of physicians' license to practice due to professional conduct, competence or substance abuse. However, the rigor of implementation of this rule is likely to be inconsistent because licensing procedures are inherently within the jurisdiction of individual states. Finally, under the Act, NPDB also receives data regarding professional review actions at hospitals and medical societies resulting in the restriction of practice (usually as hospital staff) privileges for more than 30 days, if at issue were professional conduct or competence potentially affecting patient welfare. The potency of this information is enhanced by the fact that hospitals are mandated by the federal regulation to query the NPDB for relevant data before hiring or granting privileges to a physician. In fact, there is a legal presumption that the absence of such queries indicates that the hospital had all the relevant, including all negative, information about the physician, hence the hospital become jointly liable in a medical malpractice action against the physician involved. From the involved physician's point of view the contents of the NPDB may be a very serious matter. In addition to the fact that it can and will likely affect the practitioner's chances of obtaining employment hence his/her career, its contents are virtually irremovable and unalterable, barring a court order changing or removing the information, or mandating new disciplinary proceedings the outcome of which would in turn alter the contents of the database.

Before closing, it should be noted that the federal NPDB is by no means a pioneering effort in terms of inception, timing and rigor of enforcement. States have also taken their own initiative in this regard, with perhaps New York leading the way. In New York, adverse action reports have for some time been sent to the Office of Professional Discipline of the New York State Education Department which routinely forwards a copy to the State Department of Health. In fact, some of the NPDB rules have already for some time existed in relevant New York laws. Thus, Section 2803(e) of the NY Public Health Law mandates hospitals to report various negative actions against physicians to the State Department of Health. Under Section 315 of the State Insurance Law, the NY Department of Health also receives reports on financial settlements where a malpractice action was brought about by fraud, incompetence, or negligence. Additionally, Section 2805(k) of the New York Public Health Law mandates hospitals to investigate a physician's background in terms of disciplinary and malpractice actions prior to hiring or grating staff privileges to that physician.[34]

Notes

1. Morreim, E., "Cost Containment and the Standard of Medical Care", *California Law Review*, Vol. 75, 1987. Hall, M., "Malpractice Standards Under Healthcare Cost Containment", *Law and Medical Care*, Vol. 17, 1989. Rosenblatt, R., "Redefining Administrative Liability", *Health Management Quarterly*, Vol. 12, 1stQ, 1990.
2. A vivid example of that just occurred at the time of this writing in Johnson vs. New York Health and Hospital Corporation [tried during February 1996 in New York Supreme Court - opinion unpublished at the time of this writing], involving the issue of flawed hospital security procedures allegedly to have resulted in the rape and murder of a pregnant physician and her fetus in her office/laboratory on hospital premises. The Claimant was represented by one of New York City's top and most recognized trial attorneys. If there was a settlement offer, it was apparently not accepted. The case received substantial publicity, including full television coverage. All legal circles and forums that came to the attention of this writer, particularly those aired on Court TV, predicted a plaintiff's verdict, with some divergence in opinions and expectations as to the amount of the verdict. Yet, contrary to a professional legal consensus for a plaintiff's verdict, the jury came back for the defense. The high perceived probability of a verdict for any amount, i.e. **pV**, turned into zero.
3. Keeton, W., *Prosser and Keeton on Torts*, 5th ed., West Publishing Co., St. Paul, MN, pp.150-195.
4. The writer benefited in this context from conversations with H. McKillop, MD of Mount Sinai Medical Center and School. Comments made by Mitchell Grate, Esquire, an attorney active in medical malpractice litigation also helped clarify for the writer some of the issues involved in this section of the chapter. Finally, the author's own extensive courtroom experience as an economic expert in medical malpractice trials over the past twenty years also significantly contributed to the formulation of the views presented here.
5. For the former, see Hall v. Hilburn 466 So. 2nd 856 (Miss 1985); for the latter see Zintek v. Perchik 471 N.W.2d 522, 530 (Wis.C.A. 1991).
6. 42 U.S.C.A. ## 11101-52 (West Supp.1989).
7. Danzon, P., *Medical Malpractice: Theory, Evidence and Public Policy*, Harvard University Press, Cambridge, MA, 1985. See also, Danzon, P., "The Frequency and Severity of Medical Malpractice Claims: New Evidence", *Law and Contemporary Problems*, Vol. 49, 1986. Articles noting the problems of that time also appeared as "Malpractice Crisis: How It's Hurting Medical Care", *US News and World Report*, May 26, 1975; "Sorry, America Your Policy is Canceled", *Time*, March 26, 1986. See also, *Hearings on the Liability Insurance Crisis Before the Subcommittee on Economic Stabilization of the House Committee on Banking and Finance and Urban Affairs* (Parts 1 and 2), 99th Congress, 2nd Session, July 23-Oct 2, 1986; and *Hearings on Liability Insurance Availability Before the Subcommittee on Commerce, Transportation and Tourism of the House Committee on Energy and Commerce (Part 1 and 2)*, 99th Congress 2nd Sess. (Sept 19, 1985 - April 25, 1986). Doubting the seriousness of the medical malpractice problems of the time is Henderson, J. and

Eisenberg, A., "The Quiet Revolution in Product Liability: An Empirical Study of Legal Change", *UCLA Law Review*, Vol. 37, 1990.

8.   General Accounting Office, *Medical Malpractice: A Framework for Action,* February 1987.

9.   Testimony of Richard K. Willard, Assistant Attorney General, Civil Division, US Department of Justice, in *Hearings on Liability Insurance Crisis* [see note 7 above]. See also, "State Legislatures Worried About Product Liability, Survey Finds", *Liability Week*, Sept 12, 1988.

10.   Sack, K., "Thousands of Medical Errors, But Few Lawsuits, Study Shows", *New York Times,* January 29, 1990 [the article, having surveyed New York hospitals found that while tens of thousands of injuries and thousands of deaths occurred due to medical negligence every year, only a few of the victims actually file a claim]. See also Danzon, P., *Medical Malpractice* - see above; Bovjberg, "Medical Malpractice on Trial: Quality of Care is the Important Standard", *Law and Contemporary Problems,* Vol. 49, 1986 [found that even after an acceleration of claim filings, still only a relatively small proportion of the injured actually file a complaint, and only a fraction of those receive compensation]. Reflecting on frequent assertions that premiums have been escalated by many frivolous suits, the Department of Commerce, State of Minnesota, *Medical Malpractice Claim Study 1982-1987,* Minneapolis, MN, 1989, based on insurance industry submitted data, indicates that even if "frivolous" is defined broadly, no more than some 3% of premiums are paid out for such claims, and if the definition is stricter, the proportion is reduced to well under 1% per year.

11.   See Testimony given by Robert Hunter, past Federal Insurance Administrator and President, National Insurance Consumer Organization, at the *1986 Liability Insurance Crisis Hearings,* pp. 58-59 - see citation above. See also, Robinson, "The Medical Malpractice Crisis of the 1970s: A Retrospective", *Law and Contemporary Problems*, Vol. 49, 1986; and Nye, J., Gilford J. et al., "The Causes of Medical Malpractice Crisis: An Analysis of Claims Data and Insurance Company Finances", *Georgetown Law Journal,* Vol. 76, 1988. These attest to the insurance industry's own economic fluctuations by way of so-called "underwriting cycles" as the likely causes of crises and prosperity.

12.   St. Paul Fire and Marine Insurance Co., *Physicians' and Surgeons' Update 1985: A Special Report 3,* 1985 [cited in Danzon, *Medical Malpractice: Theory and Evidence,* p.57] indicated a 55% increase in claims per 100 physicians between 1980 and 1985. In a 1987 study, the AMA indicates an approximately three-fold increase in malpractice claims per 100 physicians. By 1989, significant drops in medical malpractice claims were registered in the media. Thus, *The New York Times* on June 11, 1989 reported a drop in claims in an article entitled "Costs of Medical Malpractice Drop After an 11-Year Climb". The 1988 edition of the St. Paul Fire and Marine Insurance Company's *Physicians' and Surgeons' Update* also registers a drop in the number of claims filed. Testimonies given in the *1986 Liability Insurance Crisis Hearings* by Roper, R.T. and Herman, P.J., officials and administrators of court related administrative and statistical organizations, noted that even those increases in claims which were experienced during the late 1970s and up to about 1985 were commensurate with increases in overall medical costs, followed or coincided with increases of similar proportions in the population.

13.   General Accounting Office, *Insurance: Profitability of the Medical Malpractice and General Liability Lines*, 1987; medical malpractice insurers' reserves having increased from just under $1 billion to well over $3 billion during 1984 and 1985.

14. Jost, A., "The Necessary and Proper Role of Regulation to Assure the Quality of Healthcare", *Houston Law Review*, Vol. 25, 1988. Several articles in the *New York Times* "28,000 'Doctors' Are Feared Unfit" (5/15/86), "State Medical Boards Disciplined Record Numbers of Doctors in 1985" (11/9/89), "Doctor Who Billed Millions is Cut by New York Medicaid" (11/6/89), "Doctor Gives Up Medical License in Face of 'Love Surgery' Hearings" (1/27/89), "Jury Deliberates Fate of Physician Who Admits Killing Wife in Fight" (10/27/86), "9 Deaths Studied in Doctor's Case" (12/3/87). See also, "Army Had Evidence on Doctor Accused of Sodomy", *Washington Post*, 12/7/85, and "Doctor Sued 14 Times But No State Hearing", *Chicago Tribune* (5/10/82). Further see, *Medical Malpractice Hearings on H.R. 5110 Before the Subcommittee on Health and the Environment of the House Energy and Commerce Committee*, 99th Congress, 2nd Session 1986.

15. Department of Health and Human Services, Office of the Inspector General, Office of Analysis and Inspections, *Medical Licensure and Discipline: An Overview*, 1986. Comment, "The Healthcare Quality Improvement Act of 1986: Will Physicians Find Peer Review More Inviting?", *Virginia Law Review*, Vol. 74, 1988. Rosenberg, J., "How Bad Doctors Dodge Discipline", *Medical Economics*, 3/18/1985. Waxman, A., "Sounding Board: Medical Malpractice and Quality of Care", *New England Journal of Medicine*, Vol. 316, 1986. Comment "Physician, Heal Thyself: Because the Cure, the Health Care Quality Improvement Act May be Worse than the Disease", *Catholic University Law Review*, Vol. 37, 1988. See also, GAO, *Expanded Federal Authority Needed to Protect Medicare and Medicaid Patients From Health Practitioners Who Lose Their Licenses*, 1984.

16. The Federation of State Medical Boards of the US Inc. Exchange, 1986. *Hearing Report No. 903*, 99th Congress, 2nd Session 1986, reprinted in 1986 *US Code Congressional and Administrative News* 6384, 6385 (accompanied the HCQIA). Derbishyre, R., "Medical Licensure and Discipline in the United States" 13 (1969), cited in *Physician Heal Thyself*, noted earlier.

17. DHHS, Office of Inspector General, Office of Analysis and Inspections, *Medical Licensure and Discipline: An Overview* 16, 1986. See also, Library of Congress, Congressional Research Service, *Compilation of State Statutes on What Constitutes Unprofessional Physician Conduct*, 1986.

18. See Miller v. Eisenhower Medical Center 166 CalRptrs 826, 614 P.2d 258 (1980); Halberstadt v. Kissane 273 N.Y.S 2d 601 (1966); Jacobs v. Martin 20 NJ Super.531, 90 A.2d 151 (1982); Maimon v Sisters of Third Order 142 Ill. App. 3d 306, 96 Ill Dec 500 491 N.E. 2d (1986); McMorris v. Williamsport Hospital 597 F. Supp. 899 (M.D. Pa 1984).

19. Testimony of M.C. Faray on October 9-10, 1986 at *Hearings on H.R. 5540, The Health Care Quality Improvement Act of 1986*, Subcommittee on Civil and Constitutional Rights of the House Committee on the Judiciary, 99th Congress 2nd Session 75.

20. The following chapter will examine in detail the antitrust scene in which healthcare quality related issues are dealt with.

21. HR 4390, 99th Congress, 2nd Sess.

22. Patrick v. Burget, 800 F.2d 1498

23. 486 US 94; see also Parker v. Brown 317 US 341 (1943) which set up rigorous standards for the application of state action immunity, standards which, in view of the Supreme Court, Patrick v. Burget did not pass.

24. Statement by Congressman Wyden, 132 Cong. Rec. E735 (March 12, 1986).

25. There was an initial minimum of $35,000 as to payments, but that minimum was dropped in later revisions and was omitted from the final version of the Act.

26.   99th Congress, 2nd Session (June 26, 1986).
27.   99th Congress, 2nd Session (September 17, 1986).
28.   Ibid. # 102.
29.   Ibid. # 301(9).
30.   Title IV, Public Law 99-660; 132 Cong Rec. S17348 (October 18, 1986); 42 USC 1111-1152.
31.   NPDB is operated by UNISYS Corporation under contract with USDHHS, Division of Quality Assurance and Liability Management with annual budget during the early to mid-1990s of around $15-$20 million dollars.
32.   42 USC 1320(a).
33.   US Department of Health and Human Services. *National Practitioners Data Bank Guidebook Supplement: A Reference for Individuals and Entities Reporting to and Querying the Data Bank*, USDHHS, Public Health Service, Health Resources and Services Administration, Rockville, MD, 1990. See also, US. Department of Health and Human Services. *National Practitioners Data Bank Guidebook: Current References for Data Bank Users Individuals and Entities Reporting to and Querying the Data Bank*, USDHHS, Bureau of Health Professions, Health Resources and Services Administration, Rockville, MD, 1992.
34.   Commentary, "Observations on the National Practitioner Data Bank", *New York State Journal of Medicine*, January 1992.

12 The Legal Environment for Healthcare Quality: Competition Enforcement

At the time of this writing, Congress just passed a healthcare reform of a sort the provisions of which include care coverage portability while precluding exclusions for pre-existing conditions. In fact, healthcare reform proposals and some implemented reforms abound in the history of US healthcare policy. Some of these reforms, such as the ones currently implemented, tend to have a significant social value with a relatively insignificant impact on the severity of competition in the healthcare marketplace. Other reforms and reform proposals, however, were seen as much more significant for the healthcare *markets*, setting in motions countervailing powers from one interest group or another. In general, an important element of these countervailing powers relied on care quality. That is, how will or would the proposed or implemented healthcare reforms impact upon care quality? When it came to reforms or proposals impacting upon the structure and regulation of healthcare markets, one interest group that always became notable is that composed of the physicians themselves. Physicians always see themselves as the primary determinants of healthcare quality, and as those who are most eminently qualified to measure healthcare quality and set its appropriate level in any care environment. Typically, however, physician groups have often identified care quality almost solely in terms of the degree of autonomy which they enjoyed, or needed, to practice medicine. Thus, to the extent that this autonomy was to be infringed upon, so was the quality of care expected to decline, or at least so perceived[1].

Similar concerns have typically been expressed when competition enforcement in healthcare markets has relatively recently come to the forefront of healthcare politics and health economics. Until as recently as about 20 years ago, competitive market pressures in medicine were little known and even less concerned with phenomena. The enforcement and regulation of competition was absent, although sporadic regulation of specific elements of medical performance in designated market segments was practiced. An area of regulation was licensing of practitioners, perhaps the only one at that time that targeted the individuals. Most other regulatory efforts were aimed at hospitals, controlling their facilities and the volume of their services with the social responsibility for the cost of care in mind[2]. Antitrust and competition enforcement were for many years of no concern to the private practitioner or the hospital. If any efforts in this regard could be found, they were mainly self-imposed and voluntary, leaving many healthcare markets and economic practices within those markets vulnerable to the utmost degree to antitrust enforcement, once that enforcement were to begin. Healthcare market fruits have ripened for the antitrust pickers, the stakes became high, and the rewards tempting. However, as we will note, the defenses to most antitrust attacks involved at least a reference to if not complete reliance upon the impact of the conduct, or its denial, on the quality of care involved.

Antitrust concerns were raised in a variety of situations. Physicians complained of being denied hospital privileges. So did midwives and chiropractors. Hospitals consummated exclusive contracts with certain provider groups to perform specialized services, excluding others who could also perform those services. Hospitals agree as to division of services and specialization, e.g. burn units, emergency facilities, and so forth. Individual providers collude so as to resist third-party payers' efforts to reduce costs, or as to the minimum amount of reimbursement they would accept for various services from those payers. Hospital would be denied accreditation, or the issuance of a certificate-of-need, by an agency relying on the opinion of competing hospitals, or a physician would be denied licensing or certification by a body made of competing physicians. The list could continue to include a variety of other situations that will be touched upon later in the chapter[3]. The quality of care notion often took a prominent seat as justification for the position of one side or the other in these controversies. Thus, greater third-party reimbursement was requested to maintain quality, or the exclusion of incompetent physicians were seen as necessary to sustain care quality. These postures, however, can have at least two dimensions. The preclusion of a competing physician, if the latter is incompetent, would improve the quality of care or would at least prevent its decline, notwithstanding the fact that it would restraint competition as well. Few would doubt or debate the priority of major improvements in healthcare quality over the preservation of competition, if they do need to represent a trade-off. The preclusion of a competent provider, however, would clearly jeopardize care quality, as well as competition in the relevant market, in which case this trade-off is not relevant.

Furthermore, all of these assertions presuppose an appropriate definition and measurement of competition, and a concept of healthcare quality which is also clearly defined, delineated, and readily measurable with available or cost-effectively procurable data.

Thus, the circle of analyses commenced in this volume appears to have completed itself with this last substantive chapter of the book. Earlier chapters of this volume took great pain and time to discuss issues involved in defining, delineating and measuring healthcare quality. It raised more questions than generated answers because the appropriate quality of healthcare in many settings and for most patients in those settings is very difficult to delineate. In fact, in Chapter 4 we showed that product/service quality is a difficult concept to deal with even outside the realm of healthcare markets, in other industrial settings. Given these difficulties, one may search for some sort of minimum levels of quality. With a product or service, we might postulate that an absolute minimum level of quality that should be present from the consumer's point of view is that it should not harm the consumer if the product or service is consumed. Beyond that, the issues become highly subjective and at times arbitrary. They become a matter for "judgment", the favorite escape clause of those who for whatever reasons will not or are not able to deal with the relevant issues. In healthcare markets the complexity of these problems is compounded. Patients vary, along with the personality, practice patterns, and competence of their individual providers as well as the settings, technology, timing for and the stage of the implemented care. There is little agreement as to what quality means, how "curing" v. "caring" be interpreted, and how quality standards should be imposed in a multi-faceted, pluralistic, and still largely unregulated care delivery environment[4]. In addition, quality is often viewed as a feature that should include universal access to care. This, in turn, implies that unless one can find socially or politically justifiable reasons to the contrary, all should have access to the same level, standard and quality of care. What should that care be? At what cost? Who should subsidize and in what manner the cost for those who cannot afford the prescribed level of care? In other words, how should society deal with the perennial trade-offs between the cost and quality needed to provide this socially acceptable standard level of care for everyone?

These questions, and particularly a lack of adequate answers to them, render the application of care quality concepts to antitrust litigation difficult, and at least in the past, likely irrelevant. Nevertheless, in today's environment where concern for healthcare quality is increasing and has become not only a socio-political but also a profoundly economic issue with close connection to the profitability of the healthcare providers themselves, care quality must become an issue to be viewed as pertinent and essential for the antitrust judiciary, and particularly for judges who decide at the trial level on the admissibility of such data and information. It seems rational to assume in the socio-politics of today's healthcare delivery environment that judges may not want to find themselves in the position of appearing to sacrifice healthcare quality affecting possibly millions of people in the interest of some uncertain and largely unmeasured economic benefit that might accrue from the preservation of competition in any given market - even if the competition, the market, and market power were properly delineated as part of the litigation. It may be that a new query of economic dimensions should be introduced into antitrust actions that involve healthcare quality issues: a cost-benefit analysis aimed at ascertaining that the preservation or restoration of competition in some healthcare markets yields greater eco-social benefits than a claimed deterioration in healthcare quality if the plaintiff, say an excluded but incompetent physician, prevails. Clearly, issues of this nature would have to be viewed in terms of their degree of relevance and impact. An insignificant reduction of competition in some healthcare markets, even if properly shown, is a small price to pay for the preservation or enhancement of healthcare quality, even if only a relatively small proportion of the patient population would be affected; or, an insignificant increase in competition by allowing the wrong provider to prevail is not warranted if even a small proportion of the healthcare population will be adversely affected. Some reasonable balancing of the competitive and healthcare quality impact needs to be implemented, in addition to studies which are often needed healthcare antitrust actions, such as market definitions and delineations, market power measurements, and damage studies. The only damage that is actually being measured is that in dollar terms for the claimant. A restraint on competition in healthcare markets with its negative social consequences are normally implied or assumed if certain parameters are met, such as showing a common law based significant market share in a properly delineated market. Typically, economic experts in antitrust litigation involving healthcare markets have not been called upon to show the impact on healthcare quality, or even the economic consequences of a negative impact on healthcare quality. Nor has there been thus far any serious consideration given to weighing the relative importance of *economic damages* shown by the plaintiff (may be labeled as "private damages"), and the impact of the conduct complained of on society through affecting *competition* (may be called as "social impact no. 1"), those affecting *healthcare quality* (could be labeled as "social impact no. 2"), and the economic impact of any deterioration or enhancement in healthcare quality (may be called *"derivative social impact"*). Let us now take a bird's-eye view at the essentials of antitrust enforcement as they apply to healthcare markets.

Antitrust Principles in Healthcare[5]

Antitrust enforcement in healthcare is a relatively new phenomenon. Until the mid-1970s, antitrust statutes were considered largely irrelevant to the healthcare profession since the latter was thought of as basically a "non-commercial" activity that did not involve nor affect interstate commerce. Healthcare was seen as a self-regulating learned professional endeavor controlled in some respects, but not by way of competitive enforcement, largely by the states[6]. After the mid-1970s the exemption for the learned professions, including medicine, was lifted by a number of Supreme Court decisions. Federal antitrust laws became dominant over state regulatory provisions unless it was shown that what would otherwise be a federal antitrust violation was in fact the result of state policy implementation under state supervision. Thus, medicine became a concern, in fact subsequently a major concern, for federal competitive enforcement[7].

The federal antitrust laws are charged with at least maintaining the competitive status quo and securing market environments where businesses have an equal opportunity to compete and to succeed based on their ability. This notion was perhaps best stated some forty years ago as follows:

> "The Sherman Act was designed to be a comprehensive charter of economic liberty aimed at preserving free and unfettered competition as the rule of trade. It rests on the premise that the unrestrained interaction of competitive forces will yield the best allocation of our economic resources, the lowest prices, the highest quality and the greatest material progress, while at the same time providing an environment conducive to the preservation of our democratic political and social institutions. But even were that premise open to that question, the policy unequivocally laid down by the Act is competition[8].

The essence of this pronouncement is the preservation of *competition,* the competitive market environment, and not necessarily each and every, or any, individual *competitor,* regardless its talents, efficiency, or product quality. The ultimate beneficiary is society by way of participating consumers receiving quality products at fairly determined market prices. In healthcare markets, however, the otherwise often envisioned relatively simple interactions of demand and supply are complicated by a variety of factors. Thus, for instance, while in non-healthcare markets the consumer or consumers are functionally homogeneous, they are the buyers, in healthcare markets they are functionally often represented by at least two types of entities, those who actually receive the care and those who pay for that care. The former is, of course, the patient while the latter may be an employer, an insurance company, or a government agency. These circumstances may induce the consumer to demand more of care services than if they had to pay for most or all of those services, given the true cost and quality of those services. In addition, product information in healthcare markets is not as easily available or understood by patients as it would be in non-healthcare markets. Patients often accept the advice of their most trusted provider instead of making their own decisions pursuant to a selection process, such as they would engage in when procuring non-healthcare products or services. One should note, however, that while this attribute was typical of healthcare delivery systems in the past, managed care generated quality problems due to the gatekeepers' financial incentives to withhold care attracted significant attention in recent years by patients taking the initiative through formal complaints or even medical malpractice law suits. In other words, while technically still not trained, patients have become more sophisticated and sensitive to the quality of care they receive or should have received but were denied. Also, healthcare markets have been tempered with by some barriers to entry through provider licensing, and through regulatory measures such as certificate-of-need programs so long as they were in effect. Finally, since wide or universal access to care of some standard and quality is a sensitive social and political issue, policies aimed at the implementation of such access interferes with the market process by not allowing care to be distributed through the market's pricing mechanism but rather in response to socially cross-subsidized needs.

Notwithstanding these and some other healthcare market inhibitors, competition has become an important operational and policy factor. Purchasers are more sophisticated than ever. They use group purchasing power and hired expertise to assess care in terms of its cost and quality. The number and types of healthcare providers, particularly on the institutional scene, proliferated to unprecedented levels. So did pricing structures, service categories, and attainable quality standards. Regulatory measures, especially through the implementation of the DRG and RBRVS provider payment systems lead to serious cost containment efforts and occupancy reductions at hospitals. Third-party payers, insurance companies, managed care organizations and other entities with considerable group purchasing power extracted significant discounts from providers, particularly from hospitals, and imposed strict utilization control measures. In response, hospitals began to advertise aggressively for patients, and are attempting to recruit physicians who are most likely to attract additional patients.

Recent years also witnessed fundamental structural changes in healthcare markets. Free-standing care facilities such as emergency and urgent care clinics, birthing centers, one-day surgery facilities, and other on-site virtually shopping-center or store-front based clinics competing with hospital emergency room facilities changes the hospitals' playing fields. Physicians' access to capital facilities and equipment which in the past were available only at hospitals has also been increased. In addition, the scope and location of physicians' functions has considerably expanded due to the fact that changes in medical technology now allows the performance of many procedures in these free-standing facilities which in the past could only be performed in inpatient hospital environments. This created a multilateral competitive marketplace where free-standing clinics compete with hospitals, physicians in their own offices compete with free-standing clinics, and due to the expanded facilities at these clinics, physicians compete with those at hospitals and other allied health providing institutions such as nursing homes, long-term care, and home care facilities. Healthcare services have become unbundled both institutionally and functionally creating markets and submarkets that may be as ripe for competition as many non-healthcare markets.

Federal antitrust enforcement efforts have by far constituted the bulk of antitrust history both within and outside the healthcare field. We will review some of the key issues involved in these enforcement efforts with respect to healthcare markets. However, it should be noted that state antitrust enforcement authorities have also been active[9]. Also, the Multistate Antitrust Task Force formed in 1983 by the National Association of Attorney Generals [NAAG] includes a working group on healthcare. This gives individual states the option to proceed in antitrust actions under its state or federal law, and also two or more states to engage in interstate joint antitrust actions by way of relevant investigations and joint actions filed in federal court. In addition, an Executive Working Group on Antitrust has been formed in 1989 by the Antitrust Division, the FTC and the NAAG. They meet several times a year, and healthcare issues have been a major preoccupation.

As indicated earlier, federal enforcement was the mainstay of antitrust activity in the US for the past century, and an area of preoccupation has been with horizontal conduct restraints, or conspiracies, under Section 1 of the Sherman Act[10]. For it to be relevant, the conspiracy, whether overtly or covertly committed to a common scheme, would either need to have an anti-competitive purpose or an unreasonable or substantially anticompetitive effect[11]. If the conduct is anticompetitive with significant procompetitive elements, a *rule of reason* approach is applied weighing the procompetitive against the competitive effects with a view to determining the nature and extent of some net social effect. Thus, issues involving exclusive hospital contracts with physicians that foreclose other physicians, or the restriction of staff privileges, may be justified by various socio-economic purposes based on economies of scale or projected positive impact on care quality, hence would need to be evaluated under the rule of reason in order to determine the degree of negative impact, if any, on competition[12]. A classical statement of the essence of the *rule of reason* was put on the record some eighty years ago as follows:

> "Every agreement concerning trade, every regulation of trade, restrains. To bind, to restrain, is their very essence. The true test of legality is whether the restraint imposed is such as merely regulates and perhaps thereby promotes competition or whether it is such as may suppress or even destroy competition. To determine that question, the court must ordinarily consider the facts peculiar to the business to which the restraint is applied; its condition before and after the restraint was imposed; the nature of the restraint and its effect, actual or probable. The history of restraint, the evil believed to exist, the reason for adopting a particular remedy, the purpose or end sought to be attained, are all relevant facts"[13].

Healthcare cases in this regard were typically scrutinized in terms of the presence of anticompetitive intents by way of removing or dimuning a competitor in the relevant market, the extent of the impact on market competition, care quality, pricing, and care availability[14].

Some restraints are viewed as "unforgivable" under any set of circumstances. These are analyzed under the *per se* rule which essentially disregards the nature, purpose or the effect of an agreement and presumes conclusively that the practice constitutes a blatant restrain on competition as an automatic violation of the Sherman Act, making further inquiries redundant. *Northern Pacific* defined *per se* practices as follows:

"...There are certain agreements or practices which because of their pernicious effect on competition and lack of any redeeming virtue are conclusively presumed to be unreasonable and therefore illegal without any elaborate inquiry as to the precise harm they have caused or the business excuse for their use. This principle of *per se* unreasonableness not only makes the type of restraint which are proscribed by Sherman more certain to the benefit of everyone concerned, but it also avoids the necessity for an incredibly complicated and prolonged economic investigation into the entire history of the industry involved, as well as related industries, in an effort to determine at large whether a particular restraint was reasonable - an inquiry so often wholly fruitless when undertaken"[15].

Thus, it is the agreement itself, even if never implemented, constitutes the violation. In enforcement history, typically the following types of agreement were viewed as *per se* antitrust violations: price fixing, horizontal market allocations, group boycotts, and tying agreements[16]. The Federal Trade Commission has in more recent years applied the so-called "inherently suspect" or "*truncated rule of reason*" standards in cases where a practice is likely to restrict output and reduce competition without the presence or recognition of any significant and valid *efficiency* justification[17].

Pivotal concepts in many antitrust cases that do *not* involve *per se* conduct are the *relevant market* and *market power*[18]. Both of these point to the existence and extent of competitive restraint. They are yardsticks that essentially attempt to pinpoint the locale and the extent of competitive restraints. Significant competitive restraints in the relevant market are measured in terms of the conduct's impact on the flow of goods in the relevant market and on the geographical area that is thought to be involved. Thus, once delineated, a relevant market has product and geographical dimensions. All goods or services that display a high cross-elasticity of demand, that is, a high degree of interchangeability in the perception of relevant consumers (i.e. substitutes within comparable price ranges) belong in the same *product* market. Thus, a group ("cluster") of hospital acute care inpatient services would be defined as a relevant product market for hospitals, and speciality or sub-speciality lines for individual physician practices. A relevant healthcare product market may even be defined in the more general terms of healthcare financing if the subject of the dispute involves HMOs, insurers, and other third-party payers or reimbursers[19].

The *geographical* market dimension on the other hand looks at the community, group of communities, or region where the competitive drama is thought to play out - that is, where the claimant *and* the defendant encounter significant competition in terms of their delineated product or service. The data pertinent to geographical markets in healthcare matters are normally generated from statistics that reflect on patient flows and physician admitting patterns. In general, a key question refers to the distance that patients are willing to migrate to seek care in response to some significant price changes. In other words, in the same geographical market, patients will likely choose one hospital over another in order the procure care of a given quality at a lower price. Patient flow statistics help to delineate the geographical area(s) (cities, counties, etc.) from where providers receive most of their patient census. Queries per delineated care items (i.e. product markets) that normally need to be dealt with refer to the proportion of hospital(s') admissions from specific geographical area(s), the proportion of patients in those geographical areas seeking the delineated care items going to the hospital(s) involved, and hospital groups to which their staff providers and other physicians tend to admit patients for the indicated care items[20].

Upon delineation of the relevant product and geographical markets, attempts are made to measure the defendant(s') *market power* in order to postulate whether or not even if the conduct has occurred could there have been a significant restraint on competition. In other words, what is the extent, if any, of the social harm? In a generic sense, market power is possessed by a firm in its market if by way of its output related decisions it has a significant impact on price, and can exclude or substantially influence competition. Market power and social harm are thus inferred from the existence of market share, with the latter being expressed in terms of some controlled proportion of the market. The controlling percentage of total sales, net shipments, or in healthcare cases patient/procedure-count and related variables, often varied case-by-case, but in general constituted a majority of the market, likely at or above 60%-65%[21]. In addition to market share, courts have considered several circumstantial variables such as technological superiority, relative size of the defendant, pricing practices and price trend, and, perhaps most significantly, the presence or absence of entry barriers, for market power assessments[22].

Some Application Specifics of Antitrust Enforcement in Healthcare Markets

There is a broad range of market structure and conduct issues in healthcare that may be relevant for antitrust enforcement. These could be grouped into three categories: (a) essentially *non-price based horizontal conduct restraints,* such as joint ventures, mergers and acquisitions, organized group purchasing, shared services, coordination through alternative delivery systems, and professional associations; (b) horizontal conduct *restraint with respect to price,* such as price fixing, organized peer reviews of fees, fee surveys and information swapping, physician-hospital pricing contracts, and price discrimination; (c) *staffing issues,* such as medical staff peer reviews, exclusive contracts, constraints on allied health professionals, and hospital closed staff policies with respect to certain specialities or the entire hospital.

Increasing focus on healthcare cost containment and intensifying competitive pressures in healthcare markets prompted providers to implement certain self-protecting as well as mutually self-preserving measures. A group of these measures involves horizontal agreements among provider competitors that entails cooperation and collaboration tantamount to lessening or eliminating competition in some segments of the healthcare market. A type of horizontal conduct that clearly eliminates competition between the participants in the product line involved is a *joint venture* where the participants pool their capital, integrate operation, and share the risks in a venture that alone they could not have or would not have entered into. The alternative would be for the firms to engage in competition with the respect to the product/service involved. In some cases, such an arrangement may serve the legitimate purpose of pooling capital for producing a product/service and entering into a market as an additional competitor where the participants alone could not have had the resources to enter. However, this arrangement may also be designed simply to restrain competition between two entities. Factors such as efficiencies achieved by the arrangement along with its original purpose normally help assessing these issues. Hospitals have entered into joint venture agreements with other providers to operate facilities or to provide services. These have included ambulatory care facilities, HMOs, long-term care facilities, imaging centers, cancer screening clinics, home health agencies, and so forth. Joint ventures among physicians have been aimed at selling diagnostic or therapeutic equipment or the equipment's services, such as MRI's to patients[23]. In addition to their competitive implications, these arrangements have also raised issues on conflict of interest and fraud for the provider particularly under the Medicare and Medicaid programs[24].

Section 7 of the Clayton Act[25] proscribes anticompetitive acquisitions. The US Department of Justice - FTC joint Merger Guidelines of 1992 indicates a scrutiny of mergers in terms of the degree of relevant market concentration, the position of the parties to the venture in their market(s), entry barriers (or a lack thereof) into the market for the ventured product or service, and whether or not, barring the venture arrangement, the parties to the venture would have entered into the market by themselves as separate competitors[26]. If the parties to the venture also operate separately and competitively on their own, Sections 1 and 2 of the Sherman Act[27] may also become relevant[28].

Transactions similar to joint ventures, *mergers and acquisitions*, are also examined under Clayton 7. The Act specifically proscribes these transaction where they may result in a substantial lessening of competition in any product or geographical market, whether the parties are for-profit or not for-profit organizations, and particularly in healthcare markets where the merger is likely to inhibit cost-containment efforts through competitive restraints[29]. The economic literature and the relevant antitrust cases typically place mergers in three different categories based upon the relationship that the parties to the merger had prior to the transaction: horizontal, vertical, and conglomerate. Horizontal mergers involve prior competitors, hence inherently a lessening of competition, the extent of lessening, and its relevance for antitrust, depending on the pre-merger market shares of the merging parties. In a vertical merger the parties were in a "vertical" relationship with each other prior to the transaction, that is, at different stages of a given production process (e.g. manufacturer, wholesaler, jobber, retailer). Parties to a conglomerate merger come from different totally different often unrelated markets in terms of product or geography. Thus, these mergers are often subcategorized into product extension, market extension, and pure conglomerate mergers, depending upon what and where the parties produced prior to the merger[30].

The 1992 UDJ-FTC merger guidelines use a five dimensional analysis to determine the impact of the merger on market power. Relevant market concentration, potential competitive impact, entry conditions, merger generated efficiencies, and the financial condition of either of the merging parties in terms of whether they may be considered as "failing". Market concentration, and post-merger changes in it, are measured by the Herfindhal-Hirschman Inded (HHI), which is the sum of the squares of each firm's market share in the relevant market. Typically, with an HHI<1000 the market is deemed unconcentrated, moderate concentration is suggested by 1000<HHI<1800, and, from a competitive point of view, notably high concentration is indicated if HHI>1800. If the merger increases the HHI by 150 points in moderately and highly concentrated markets respectively, policy intervention may be called for by the Guidelines. Thus, whether or not mergers in healthcare markets will attract antitrust attention depends, among other factors, on the relevant market and the merger parties' market share. Hospital mergers in large metropolitan areas with many other hospitals are less likely to get attention than those in small communities or rural regions with a few hospitals. However, the merger of two hospitals even in metropolitan areas may be of significance if the relevant product is such (e.g. highly specialized tertiary care, cardiac or neurosurgery) that the parties to the merger are significant players in that relevant product market, within the geographical market of the metropolitan area. In addition, if the merger was likely to increase prices or restrict output to third-party payers, policy intervention was also called for[31].

Organized *group purchasing,* another non-price related horizontal conduct restraint, is actually a joint venture of limited scope prompted by competitive pressures to economize. The group normally succeeds in getting price concessions from suppliers in return for contracted volume purchases. However, while it may be an effective vehicle to reduce costs, it may also harbor socially objectionable anti-competitive efforts, or may be seen as such by those who are excluded from the group either as members or accessed suppliers both claiming group boycotts. Furthermore, the extracted price differential may also be seen as price discrimination under Section 2 of the Clayton Act as amended by the Robinson-Patman Act, or attempts to monopolize under Section 2 of the Sherman Act[32]. In general, the competitive impact of these practices depends on a number of factors. In addition to the basic motive for forming the group - i.e. cost reduction or competition foreclosure, these include the degree to which non-member providers or suppliers also have access to terms included in the groups contract, the actual and potential market power of the group, whether or not members have access to suppliers outside the group, can all suppliers bid openly for the contract, length of the contract term, and the criteria for choosing suppliers. *Shared service/equipment* arrangements are, in terms of their competitive concerns and consequences, similar to group purchasing organizations, and may also be viewed as joint ventures of a sort. Providers jointly purchase or share equipment or services. These services include non-medical ones such as computer services, billing and collections, and purchasing, and medical ones such as blood banks, clinical facilities and laboratory services may also be shared. Several hospitals may operate only one radiology department, or jointly buy and utilize MRI equipment. Once again, the factors to be weighed and the issues to be considered in order to determine competitive restraints, if any, are similar to those mentioned before in connection group purchasing organizations. In particular, agreements as to the price at which the shared services are sold to patients or non-participating providers, if the parties to the agreements exclude other providers, or if the agreements involve some sort of market division, social concerns and antitrust attention would likely be aroused[33].

In response to competitive pressures and cost containment efforts, *managed care systems* have proliferated in recent years. The establishment of HMOs, PPOs, IPAs, and so forth have, in fact, been encouraged by public officials as a way to cope with spiraling costs and to make healthcare accessible on a wider scale and at a more reasonable price. Managed care organizations were also seen as aggressive competitive catalysts in healthcare markets[34]. These organizations may be formed by any enterprising people with proper capital and expertise, but are normally established by insurance companies and other third party-payers, employers, hospitals and other providers, and other independent entities. They may be a source for social concern and antitrust attention, particularly if healthcare providers are involved in their establishment. Issues such as monopolization or attempts to monopolize, exclusive contracts, price fixing, and concerted refusals to deal, arose pursuant to managed care operations[35]. In cases of non-provider established managed care organizations, physicians conspired not deal with, group boycott, managed care solicitation for service in order to resist lower prices and reduced physician income, and hospitals refused to provide staff privileges for managed care affiliated physicians. In general, it appears that within the context of healthcare market competition the key issues in managed care environments point to provider fee setting mechanisms and, just as importantly, provider engagement and participation policies[36].

Trade association issues date far back in antitrust history[37]. Healthcare providers of all types belong to professional associations which represent their interests, disseminate information and data of common concern, and in general function as a forum and communication center. However, by definition, many members of these associations are actual or potential competitors of each other to various degrees depending upon their geographical location and specialities. While they would normally not discuss prices and fees directly outside the confines of association meetings, these and related items of information could be exchanged through the means and media of the association. The association could act as an instrument of competitive restraint. In general, the role of professional associations is socially questionable and may merit antitrust scrutiny if it functions as a forum for setting prices or transaction terms, restricts competition by fair advertising, limits association membership in bad faith, and all this along with the association through its members possessing significant market power[38].

Price related horizontal conduct in healthcare has been the focus of antitrust enforcement since the mid-1970s when competition in medical markets came under social scrutiny. *Price fixing*, normally understood to be any type of interference or meddling with the market's pricing mechanism regardless its outcome and effect on prices, has been perhaps the single most notorious policy target[39]. The case that is perhaps most often cited in connection with price fixing and price related anti-competitive issues in medicine was played out in Arizona[40]. Attempting to deal with existing third-party payer systems, two medical foundations tried to promote and coordinate traditional fee-for-service alternatives by way of proposed fee schedules. In spite of the fact that the fee schedules served cost containment principles by being reasonable, that they were proposed and voluntary, that participating physicians could also partake in other plans, the Court found the arrangement a *per se* violation of the Sherman Act. A vertical form of price fixing, or at least its appearance, may be found in situations where otherwise independent physicians (radiologists, pathologists, anesthesiologists) abide by a hospital's requests regarding the pricing of their services simply because they happened to be based at that hospital[41].

The Health Care Quality Improvement Act, discussed in the previous chapter, provides antitrust immunity to professional peer reviewers if the review is aimed at provider competence in service. It does not appear to cover peer reviews of professional fees, whether such fees are usual, customary and reasonable, or if the services performed were medically essential or necessary. Given that peer review committees are normally staffed by competing physicians, price oriented peer reviews could be a basis for fee arrangements, or a source of information to implement some sort of price fixing scenario that could lead to price stabilization or forestall price competition that would have otherwise taken place[42].

A third general and historically perhaps the most dominant application specific for antitrust enforcement in healthcare is related to *staffing* issues such as peer performance reviews, exclusive contract, and closed hospital environments. While enforcement agencies tend to consider peer reviews pro-rather than anti-competitive, physicians who are adversely affected by a review often turn to litigation under some theory of competitive restraint to seek remedy to which they feel entitled[43]. The issues typically center on denial of staff membership applications, unfavorable alterations of previous staff relations, foreclosure of some physicians by exclusive contracts with others, foreclosure of allied health personnel (podiatrists, chiropractors, etc.), and partial or complete closings of medical staff. The anti-competitive substance of these issues centers on conspiracies, specifically conspiracies to boycott the claimant. Conspiracies may be alleged between the hospital and its entire medical staff, the hospital and individual physicians on staff, and among individual staff members. While, in general, an institution and its personnel are considered to be a single entity incapable of conspiring among themselves if members of the personnel have no private interest (over and beyond that of the institution) in the conspiracy or its outcome[44], hospitals and their *medical staff* (not hospital employees), and have been typically viewed as having substantial diverging economic interests and, therefore, capable of a conspiracy[45].

Before taking a closer look as to how care quality issues were approached in antitrust, a brief recount of some of the major categories of *antitrust defenses* in healthcare is in order. First, the *Health Care Quality Improvement Act*'s immunity provisions has been discussed at length in the previous chapter. Thus, we will not deal with it again here. *Nonprofit* hospitals have attempted to claim immunity based on the provision within the FTC Act which appears to limit the FTC's jurisdiction to those firms "organized to carry on business for its own profit or that of its members"[46]. The FTC and the courts have typically viewed non-profit hospitals as functioning for the benefit and profit of its members. Mergers among non-profit hospitals have been systematically scrutinized by the FTC[47]. Some thought that the passage of the 1974 National Health Planning and Resources Development Act, designed to augment healthcare cost containment efforts and to coordinate health planning at state, local and federal levels, may render healthcare firms immune from antitrust scrutiny. However, the so called *implied repeal of the antitrust laws* defense did not apply, even before the Act was repealed · in 1986[48]. Attempts were made to invoke another defense, *business of insurance under the McCarran-Ferguson Act,*[49] in some healthcare matters. The practices relevant to this exemption need to relate to state law, normally do not apply to acts of conspiracy to boycott, coerce or intimidate, and must involve taking or spreading of risk, without being preoccupied with cost-containment. Thus, prepaid health policies may be viewed as the "business of insurance" to the extent that the policy underwrites risks instead of just being a vehicle for healthcare procurement[50]. Also, the 1984 *Local Government Antitrust Act* protects local governments or their officials and employees against antitrust damages, though not against injunctive relief, if they were acting in their official capacity[51]. A similar defense directed at state actions ("*state action doctrine*") was predicated upon the notion that the antitrust laws were not intended to apply to the conduct of state governments, or to conduct that was undertaken upon the state's request on behalf of the state, or to conduct that was undertaken under the direct supervision and active control of the state. However, this defense was almost consistently found to be irrelevant to hospital mergers and in most provider review processes.

Finally, for federal antitrust laws to be relevant to alleged conduct, it must be shown that the conduct took place in, or significantly affected, *interstate commerce*. Otherwise, relevant state antitrust statutes may apply. For some time, this has been a convenient defense in hospital staff privilege claims. However, since the early 1990s, the denial of staff privilege even to a single physician generated arguments that interstate commerce was affected[52].

Healthcare Quality in Antitrust - A Closer Look

A brief review of some of the antitrust decisions that pertain to professional services, including medicine, does not seem to indicate that the courts have been particularly preoccupied with quality, including healthcare quality, issues. In fact, it appears that in general little more than lip-service was paid to the issue. Antitrust cases in healthcare, as they have been in other sectors of the economy for the past century, continued to emphasize social goals and benefits for the consumer, to be attained by productive and allocative efficiencies. The latter in turn are thought to be enhanced directly with the preservation, or increase, in market competition. Yet, care quality issues can play an important role in antitrust litigation, in spite of the fact that Congress, when enacting the antitrust statutes, clearly meant to protect not even so much the competitor but rather competition, as source of productive and allocative efficiencies, in the interest of society as a whole. Let us examine a scenario, hypothetical as it may be, illustrative of the role that the notion of care quality could play, along with issues relating to competition and efficiency. Let us assume that a care policy making organization, say the

College of Anesthesiologists (COA), mandates that its members cannot work or professionally associate with nurse anesthetists, and that its members can not serve as staff at hospitals that also extend staff privileges to nurse anesthetists. Conventional antitrust theory would suggests that this policy and practice substantially restrains competition in the product market for anesthesiological services and in the relevant geographical market, whatever the latter happened to be. COA, on the other hand, could forcefully argue that the policy was designed and implemented to protect the patient by at least securing and more likely enhancing healthcare quality in the operating rooms. Hypothetically, the College could introduce data and information to the effect that using nurse anesthetists increases the risk of injury and death to anaesthetized patients in the operating rooms, showing for instance that in surgical procedures performed under general anesthesia more patients suffered brain damage or died due to anesthesiological malfeasance when administered by nurses than when the patient was managed during the procedure by a board certified anesthesiologists. Clearly, the issue would then be whether or not this evidence is relevant to the antitrust aspects of the case. Is care quality, whatever level of it, essential for competition? Does it serve competition, or is it independent from it? Is competition essential, or even a prerequisite for attaining some acceptable level of care quality? In other words, how does a quality of care defense fit into traditional antitrust litigation?

One could argue that the social benefits derived from not getting injured or killed in the operating room (with some reliable probability figure attached to such an event if nurse anesthetists are involved) far exceed the social costs of competitive restraints or some given level or significance. Obviously both sides of this inequality would need to be properly defined and measured so that their comparison is meaningful. In other words, what amount of competitive restraints in terms of their price and output effects would society be willing to tolerate in order to avoid how many deaths, and during what time period? Obviously, this question can be restated in various ways by holding one or the other element of the trade-off constant. It can be further reasoned that whatever competitive restrictions may ensue from the policy, their price and output effect, and certainly their unfavorable price effect, for the consumer is negligible because even if prices increase as output may diminish, the real value of the service will have at least remained constant and may have even increased: the higher nominal price simply reflects upon higher quality that ostensibly ensues from making operating room anesthetics the exclusive territory of MDs. It could also be argued in the hypothesis that certified MDs represent a better known service in the mind of the patients than do nurses, and in that respect the market mechanism is enhanced because better informed consumers make more rational decisions, and the information gap that often plagues consumer decisions in medical markets is mitigated. Given this argument's relative proximity to orthodox efficiency considerations, tradition bound antitrust courts would more likely listen to this latter type of argument than to arguments based on some sort of quality-competition tradeoffs. At any rate, which quality related argument is more appropriate in which particular case would clearly depend on the many dimensions of the fact situation at hand.

As I indicated earlier, the consideration of quality issues by the courts in antitrust cases appears to have been relatively meager. Before the 1975 landmark decision which cast aside the immunity of the learned professions[53], product or service quality issues in antitrust litigation were virtually non-existent, apart from the occasional lip-service to the notion by reciting the virtues of competition in terms of its positive impact on quality as well as on the rest of the market[54]. In *Goldfarb*, there was perhaps a reference to quality, but only by implation:

> "The *public service aspect* [emphasis added], and other features of the professions, may require that particular practice, which could properly be viewed as a violation of the Sherman Act in another context, be treated differently"[55].

Three years later, the Court decided a case involving professional engineers whose professional ethics, promulgated by their Society, prohibited competitive bidding in order to prevent a situation which could evolve into "... inferior work with consequent risk to public safety and health"[56]. In fact, the Society claimed that competitive bidding was likely to be harmful to public safety. So, here we see an argument *against* competition in order to serve the interest of quality, rather than the traditional line of argument that competition itself serves product/service quality. The Court, having pro-scribed the Society's practice, clearly prescribed to the traditional antitrust argument to the effect that competition comes first and all others, including quality, considerations come after:

> "... the judiciary cannot directly protect the public against [defective products that may cause injury] by conferring monopoly privileges on the manufacturers"[57].

These cases related to professional markets, but not to healthcare. Yet, healthcare markets clearly possess attributes that other commercial markets do not, attributes which cannot be found even in the professional markets discussed thus far. Thus, neither the legal nor the professional engineering markets experience significant relevance of third-party payers. In addition, in neither of these markets do the principals assume the key role of agent and advisor that physicians assume in relation to their patients in healthcare markets. Thirdly, in neither of these professional markets, nor as a matter of fact do we find in other markets the consumers' preoccupation with quality even in the face of limited knowledge to the extent that we encounter it in healthcare. Yet, even in healthcare markets, the antitrust courts' preoccupation with care quality as a significant factor for ultimate judicial decisions is very limited. In the landmark Maricopa case, cited several times earlier in this chapter, a price fixing effort was found to be a *per se* violation of the Sherman Act, but care quality did not enter into the proceedings beyond the observation by the Court that even the defendants did not resort to care quality arguments in justification for their conduct, that is, that care quality was in some way to be enhanced by the conspiracy[58]. Nor did the defendants invoke any type of care quality defense in a subsequent major healthcare antitrust decision, and, even if they did, their arguments would have very likely been swept aside by the Court's preoccupation with the traditional antitrust notions of productive and allocative efficiencies and their impact on service prices and availability[59]. The Court concluded that the defendant hospital did not violate the antitrust laws by signing an exclusive contract with one anesthesiologist thus foreclosing another anesthesiologist from having access to the hospital's facilities simply because the hospital had no significant market power in the relevant service and geographical markets. The Court found for the defendant hospital not because its exclusive contract in some ways enhanced care quality, but rather because lacking market power the hospital's conduct had no significant anti-competitive consequences for the market, notwithstanding healthcare market imperfections such as the dominance of third-party payers and the consumers' lack of adequate relevant product information for making rational choices.

In a third landmark healthcare case the defendants did explicitly include care quality as part of their argument. In fact, they relied on care quality as their primary justification for engaging in a boycott of some healthcare insurers[60]. Indiana dentists, organized through a federation, refused to supply claim forms and x-rays to a selected group of dental insurers because the latter capped payments and reimbursements to a level that was considered the lowest for "adequate treatment". The FTC found the conduct in violation of Section 5 of the FTC Act. The dentists' care quality based argument centered on the assertion that dental x-rays alone did not give the payer adequate clinical information for properly assessing the dental problems involved, and deciding whether and how much should be paid for dental services. The 7th Circuit reversed, finding essentially that whatever competitive restraints may have come about as a results of the boycott, it was not significant enough to offset the possible social benefits from a "legal, moral, and ethical policy of quality and proper dental care"[61]. Quality of care considerations seemed to have prevailed, but not for long. The Supreme Court upheld the Commission's order on the basis that no federation or other collective action has the right to withhold, on behalf of their members' customers or patients, information from payers, even if it did not increase prices. Furthermore, the defense's care quality related argument was rejected because, first, it is "non-economic", and, second

> "where there is such a divergence of professional judgment exists, the treatment recommendation made by the patient's dentist should [not necessarily] be assumed to be the one that in fact represents the best interest of the patient"[62].

The Court's view is clear. Professional activity, even if genuinely motivated by quality considerations, cannot be accepted if it significantly impacts upon market competition, pricing and output. Healthcare quality is subjective and is difficult to define as well as measure. Hence, different assertions about quality may be difficult to asses, compare and judge. A notion that this volume started with, extensively discussed in the process, and is once again forced to conclude near its end. In the context of contemporary healthcare antitrust litigation, this means that there is no single recognized defense formulated in terms of care quality alone.

Notes

1. Weller J., "Free Choice as a Restraint of Trade in American Health Care Delivery and Insurance", *Iowa Law Review*, Vol. 69, 1984
2. Certificate of Need (CON) Programs, and Medicare/Medicaid imposed restrictions and monitoring processes (such as PSROs) on hospitals were the thrust of these regulations.
3. Gross v. Memorial Hospital system 789 F.2d 353 (7th Cir. 1986). Stone v. William Beaumont Memorial Hospital 782 F.2d 609 (6th Cir. 1986). Nurse Midwifery Assoc.

v. Hibbett 549 F. Supp 1185 (MD TN 1982). Aasum v. Good Samaritan Hospital 395 F. Supp. 363 (D.Or.1975), aff'd 542 F.2d 792 (9th Cir. 1976). See also, "Note, Health Professionals' Access to Hospitals: A Retrospective and Prospective Analysis", *Vanderbilt Law Review*, Vol. 34, 1981. Wilk v. American Medical Association 719 F.2d 207 (7th Cir. 1983). Jefferson Parish Hospital District No. 2. v. Hyde 466 US 2 (q984). Kuck v. Bensen 647 F. Supp. 743 (D.Me. 1986). National Gerimedical Hospital v. and Gerontology Center v. Blue Cross of Kansas City 452 US 378 (1981). Hospital Building Co. v. Trustees of the Rex Hospital 691 F.2d 678 (4th Cir. 1982). Arizona v. Maricopa County Medical Society 457 US 332 (1982). Ratino v. Medical Service of the District of Columbia 718 F.2d 1260 (4th Cir. 1983). FTC v. Indiana Federation of Dentists 476 US 447 (1986). US v. North Dakota Hospital Association 640 F. Supp 1028 (D.N.D 1986). Kaefoot v. American College of Surgeons 652 F. Supp. 882 (N.D. Ill. 1986). St. Joseph Hospital Inc. v. Hospital Corporation of America 795 F.2d 948 (11th Cir. 1986).

4.   Some of these issues are discussed in Bovbjerg, R.R., "Competition Versus Regulation in Medical Care: An Overdrawn Dichotomy", *Vanderbilt Law Review*, Vol. 34, 1981.

5.   For a detailed expose of antitrust issues in healthcare, see Seplaki, L., *Cost and Competition in American Medicine: Theory, Policy and Institutions*, University Press of America, Lanham, MD, 1994, Part IV, Chapters 19-24.

6.   In addition to the federal antitrust laws, states (except Pennsylvania) have their own antitrust statutes which are basically patterned after the Sherman and Clayton Acts. New York and California appears to have the most comprehensive state antitrust laws in the country.

7.   Golfarb v. Virginia State Bar 421 US 773 (1975); Canto v. Detroit Edison Co. 428 US 579 (1976); Hospital Building Corp. v. Trustees of Rex Hospital 425 US 738 (1976); National Society of Professional Engineers v. US 435 US 679 (1978); Summit Health Limited v. Pinhas 111S.Ct 1842 (1991); Patrick v. Burget 486 US 94 (1988); FTC v. Indiana Federation of Dentists 476 US 447 (1986); Arizona v. Maricopa County Medical Society 457 US 332 (1982).

8.   Northern Pacific Railway Co. v. US 356 US 1 (1958) at 4-5.

9.   State of Maryland v. Blue Cross and Blue Shield Association 620 F. Supp. 907 (D.Md 1985); State of Colorado v. State of Colorado Union of Physicians and Surgeons, 1990-91 Trade Cas. (CCH) #68, 968 (D.Col. 1990); Minnesota v. Southern Minnesota Health Alliance, No. CO-90-766 (6/20/1990); New York v. Brooks Drug Inc 90 Civ. 4330 (SDNY June 30, 1990); Washington v. Wenatchee Valley Clinic, No. 88-161-AAM (3/29/1988).

10. 15 U.S.C. #1

11. Monsanto Co. v. Spray-Rite Service Corp 465 US 752 (1984); Brown v. Our Lady of Lourdes Medical Center Inc. 767 F. Supp. 618 (DNJ 1991), aff'd 961 F.2d 207 (3rd Cir. 1992).

12. Smith v. Northern Michigan Hospitals Inc. 703 F.2d 942 (6th Cir. 1983); Bahn v. NME Hospitals Inc. 929 F.2d 14040 (9th Cir.), cert denied 112 S.Ct 617 (1991).

13. Justice Brandeis in Board of Trade of City of Chicago v. US 246 US 231, at 238 . (1918).

14. Jefferson Parish Hospital District No. 2 v. Hyde 466 US 2 (1984); Quinn v. Kent General Hospital Inc. 617 F. Supp. 1226 (D.Del.1985); May v. Hospital Authority of Henry County 596 F. Supp 120 (ND Ga. 1984); Robinson v. McGovern 521 F. Supp. 842 (WD Pa. 1981); Lie v. St. Joseph Hospital of Mount Clemens 964 F.2d 567 (6th Cir. 1992).

15. Northern Pacific Railway Co. v. US 356 US 1 (1958).

16. Business Electronics Corporation v. Sharp Electronics Corp. 108 S.Ct. 1515 (1988); Arizona v. Maricopa County Medical Society 457US 332 (1982); US v. Socony Vacauum Oil Co. 310 US 150 (1940); NCAA v. Board of Regents of the University of Oklahoma 468 US 85 (1984); Bloom v. Hennepin County 783 F. Supp. 418 (D.Minn 1992); Klor's Inc v. Broadway Stores Inc 359 US 207 (1959); FTC v. Indiana Federation of Dentists 476 US 447 (1986); Wilk v. AMA 895 F.2d 352 (7th Cir. 1989); Eastman Kodak Co. v. Image Technical Services Inc. 112 S.Ct.2072 (1972), Jefferson Parish Hospital Case, see fn.14; Fortner Enrterprises Inc. v. US Steel 394 US 495 (1969).

17. Massachusetts Board of Registration in Optometry 110 FTC 549 (1988); In re Detroit Auto Dealers Association Inc. 111 FTC 47 (1989), affirmed 955 F.2d 457 (6th Cir. 1992).

18. For a detailed discussion of these concepts, refer to Seplaki, L., *Cost and Competition in American Medicine*, Part 2, Chs 7-10, and as cited in fn. 5.

19. In non-healthcare markets two of the significant major cases were US v. E.I. DuPont de Nemours & Co. 351 US 377 (1956); US v. Times Picayune Publishing Co 345 US 594 (1953). In healthcare markets, see US v. Rockford Memorial Hospital 898 F.2d 1278 (7th Cir. 1990); Jefferson Parish Hospital District - see earlier cite; Gonzales v. Insignales 1985-2 Trade Cas. (CCH) #66, 701 (ND Ga, 1985); Mays v. Hospital Authority of Henry County 596 F. Supp 120 (ND Ga 1984); Pontius v. Childrens Hospital 552 F. Supp 1352 (WD Pa. 1982); Robinson v. Magovern 521 F. Supp. 842 (WD PA. 1981); Ball Memorial Hospital Inc. v. Mutual Hospital Insurance Inc. 784 F.2d 1325 (7th Cir. 1986); US Healthcare Inc. v. US Health Resource Inc. 1992-1 Trade Cas. (CCH) #69, 697 (D.N.H. 1992).

20. In addition to fn. 19, also see US v. Carilion Health System 707 F. Supp. 840 (WD Va.); Hospital Corporation of America v. FTC 106, FTC 351 (1985) aff'd 807 F.2d 1381 (7th Cir. 1986); *In re* American Medical International Inc. 104 FTC 1 (1984)

21. See Jefferson Parish Hospital District; See also Weiss v. York Hospital 745 F.2d 786 (3rd Cir. 1984) that required at least an 80% market share; Hayden Publishing Co. v. Cox Broadcasting Corp. 730 F.2d 64 (2nd Cir. 1984), finding the possibility of monopoly power even under 50%; Reazin v. Blue Cross and Blue Shield of Kansas Inc. 899 F.2d 951 (10th Cir. 1990) saw 45%-62% market share as an indication of monopoly power; Barry v. Blue Cross of California 805 F.2d 866 (9th Cir. 1986), a 16% market share was definitely not enough; yet, in Energex Lighting Industries Inc. v. North American Philips Lighting Corp 656 F. Supp. 914 (SDNY, 1987) a 25% market share was enough to conclude that market power was present.

22. Ball Memorial Hospital Inc. v. Mutual Hospital Insurance Inc. 784 F.2d 1325 (7th Cir. 1986)

23. Hassan v. Independent Practice Associates PC 698 F. Supp. 679 (ED Mich. 1988); M&M Medical Supplies & Service Inc. v. Pleasant Valley Hospital Inc. 1992-2 Trade Cas. (CCH) #70, 059 (4th Cir. 1992) Key Enterprises of Delaware Inc. v. Venice Hospital 919 F.2d 1550 (11th Cir. 1990); Advanced Healthcare Systems Inc. v. Rador Community Hospital 910 F.2d 139 (4th Cir. 1990).

24. Note Medicare Anti-Kickback Statute 42 U.S.C. #1370(a)-76(b), and Ethics in Patient Referral Act of 1989, 42 U.C.C. ## 1395.

25. 15 U.S.C.#18

26. See US. v. Penn-Olin Chemical Co. 378 US 158 (1964). The Hard-Scott-Rodino Act, 15 U.S.C. #18a, applies to significant joint ventures as well as mergers and acquisition in terms of its pre-merger reporting requirements. These reporting requirements are mandated by way of Section 7a of the Clayton Act when (a) one of the merger parties' net revenues (or assets) exceed $100 million, with the other party's corre-

sponding values are at least $10 million, and the value of the acquired assets is over $15 million, and (b) the acquisition of securities confers control over an organization with sales or assets over 25 million.

27. 15 U.S.C. #1 and #2.

28. General Leaseways Inc. v. National Truck Leasing Association 744 F.2d 588 (7th Cir. 1988), and in healthcare, see Arizona v. Maricopa County Medical Society 457 US 332 (1982)

29. FTC v. University Health Systems Inc. 938 F.2d 1206 (11th Cir. 1991).

30. US v. Philadelphia National Bank 374 US 321 (1963); Brown Shoe Co. v. US 294 US 294 (1962) - has both horizontal and vertical attributes; FTC. v. Procter & Gamble Co. 386 US 568 (1967)

31. US v. Carilion Health Systems 707 F. Supp. 840 (WD Va. 1989); US v. Rockford Memorial Hospital 898 F.2d 1278 (7th Cir. 1990); see also FTV v. University Health Inc.

32. 15 U.S.C. 13, and 15 U.S.C. 2, respectively. See, White and White Inc. American Hospital Supply Corporation 540 F. Supp 951 (WD Mich 1982); Langston Corp. v. Standard Register Co. 553 F. Supp. 632 (ND Ga. 1982). See also, USDJ *Business Review Letter* 6/9/82 to the Ohio Hospital Association, and the FTC's Staff Advisory Opinion 4/23/1982 to the Louisiana Healthcare Association.

33. See Arizona v. Maricopa County Medical Society; White v. Rockingham Radiologists Ltd 820 F.2d 98 (4th Cir. 1987); Bernard General Hospital Inc. v. Hospital Service Association of New Orleans Inc. 712 F.2d 978 (5th Cir. 1983); Also see USDJ *Business Review Letter* 8/27/80 to Lakewood Hospital.

34. Rule, C.F. (Assistant Attorney General - USDJ), *Remarks Before the Group Health Association of America*, Washington, DC, 2/28/89. Arquit, K.J. (Director, Bureau of Competition - FTC), *Remarks Before the Chicago Bar Association,* Chicago, IL, 1/17/90.

35. See again, Arizona v. Maricopa County; also Hahn v. Oregon Physicians' Service 868 F.2d 1022 (9th Cir. 1988); PA Dental Association v. Medical Service Association of Pennsylvania 574 F. Supp. 457 (MD PA. 1983); and Ball Memorial Hospital Inc. v. Mutual Hospital Insurance Inc. 784 F.2d 1325 (7th Cir. 1986).

36. AMA v. US 317 US 519 (1943); Brown v. Mahoning Medical Society 1982-1 Trade Cas. (CCH) # 64, 557 (ND Ohio, 1982); FTC. v. Indiana Federation of Dentists 476 US 447 (1986); Rill, J.F., "Criminal Antitrust Prosecution in Healthcare: An Avoidable Prescription", Speech before the Antitrust Law Section, ABA (8/7/89); Reazin v. Blue Cross and Blue Shield of Kansas Inc. 663 F. Supp. 1360 (DC Kan. 1987); also see Blue Cross of Washington and Alaska v. Kitsap Physicians Service 1982-1 Trade Cas. #64, 589 (WD Wash. 1981); Barry v. Blue Cross of California 805 F.2d 866 (9th Cir. 1986).

37. See a brief discussion of these issues in Seplaki, L., *Antitrust and The Economics of the Market*, Harcourt, Brace, Jovanovich Inc. , San Diego, CA, 1982, Part II, Ch 4. See also, American Column & Lumber Company v. US 257 US 377 (1921); Maple Flooring Mfrs Association v. US 268 v. 563 (1925); Sugar Institute Inc. v. US 297 US 553 (1936).

38. FTC v. AMA 94 FTC 701 (1979); *In re* Massachusetts Board of Registration in Optometry 110 FTC 549 (1988); Arizona v. Maricopa County; US v. Massachusetts Allergy Sociey Inc. 1992-1 Trade Cas. (CCH) #69, 846 (D.Mass 1992); *In re* Connecticut Chiropractic Assocation 56 Fed. Reg 23586 (5/22/1991); FTC v. Broward County Medical Association 99 FTC 622 (1982); Kreuzer v. American Academy of Periodontology 735 F.2d 1479 (DDC 1984); Marrese v. American Academy of Orthopedic Surgeons 1991-1 Trade Cas. (CCH) # 69, 398.

39. For a classic definition of price fixing refer to US v. Socony-Vacuum Oil Co. 310 US 150 at p. 221 (1940).
40. Arizona v. Maricopa County Medical Society 457 US 332 (1982); se also FTC Staff Letter to the American Society of Internal Medicine (4/19/1985); US v. A. Lnoy Alston D.M.D., PC 974 F.2d 1206 (9th Cir. 1992); US v. Hospital Association of Greater DeMoines Inc. Civ. No. 4-92-70648 (SD Iowa, 1992); American College of Obstetricians and Gynecologists 88 FTC 955 (1976); Minnesota Medical Association 90 FTC 377 (1977); US v. South Carolina Health Care Association Inc. 1980-1 Trade Cas. (CCH) # 63, 316 (DSC 1980); US v. Montana Nursing Home Association Inc. 1982-2 Trade Cas. (CCH) #64, 852 (D.Mon. 1982); American Society of Internal Medicine 05 FTC 505 (1985); US v. North Dakota Hospital Association 640 F. Supp. 1028 (DND 1986); US v. Massachusetts Allergy Society Inc. 1992-1 Trade Cas. (CCH) #69, 846 (D.MA 1992); *In re* Southbank IPA Inc. 5 Trade Reg. Rep. (CCH) #23, 065 (Oct 9, 1991); US v. Burgstiner 1991-1 Trade Cas. (CCH) #69, 422 (SD Ga. 1991).
41. See Konik v. Champlain Valley Physicians Hospital Medical Center 733 F.2d 1007 (2d. Cir. 1984), and Rockland Physician Associates PC. v. Grodin 616. Supp. 945 (SDNY 1985).
42. These issues were covered in Ratino v. Medical Service of District of Columbia 718 F.2d 1260 (1983); *FTC Staff Advisory Opinions* to - Iowa Dental Association (4/3/83), American Podiatry Association (8/18/1983), National Capital Area Society of Plastic and Reconstructive Surgeons (4/23/91). See also issues involving third-party payers with significant provider control in Addino v. Genesee Valley Medical Care Inc. 593 F. Supp. 892 (WDNY 1984); Glen Eden Hospital Inc. v. Blue Cross and Blue Shield of Michigan Inc. 740 F.2d 423 (6th Cir. 1984), and FTC, *Enforcement Policy Regarding Physician Agreements to Control Medical Prepayment Plans,* 46 Fed. Reg. 48, 982 (10/5/1991).
43. See Rule C. Assistant Atty General USDJ. Letter to the American Medical Association (12/26/86), and Arquit, K.J. Director, Bureau of Competition Federal Trade Commission "New Concern in Health Care Antitrust Enforcement: Acquisition and Exercise of Market Power by Physician Ancillary Joint Ventures", Remarks Before the National Health Lawyers Association (1/30/1992).
44. See Harvey v. Fearless Ferris Wholesale Inc. 589 F.2d 451 (9th Cir. 1979); H&B Equipment Company v. International Harvester Co. 577 F.2d 239 (5th Cir. 1978); Oksanen v. Page Memorial Hospital 945 F.2d 696 (4th Cir. 1991).
45. Oltz v. St. Peters Community Hospital 861 F.2d 1440 (9th Cir. 1988); Weiss v. New York Hospital 745 F.2d 814 (3rd Cir. 1984); Todorov v. DCH Healthcare Authority 921 F.2d 1438 (11th Cir. 1991).
46. 115 USC #44.
47. See, AMA v. FTC. 638 F.2d 443 (2nd Cir. 1992); US v. Rockford Memorial Corp. 898 F.2d 1278 (7th Cir. 1990); Adventist Health System/West and Ukiah Adventist Hospital, 5 Trade Reg. Rep. (CCH) #23038 (8/2/1991); FTC v. University Health Inc. 938 F.2d 1206 (11th Cir. 1991).
48. See *National Health Planning and Resources Development Act of 1974,* Pub.L. No. 93-641, 88 Stat. 2225. Repealed by Health Programs, Pub. L. No. 99-660, 100 Stat. 3743. See also National Gerimedical Hospital and Gerontology Center v. Blue Cross of Kansas City 452 US 378 (1981); FTC v. American Medical International Inc. 104 FTC 1 Trade Reg. Rep (CCH) #22, 170 (1984); Boulware v. State of Nevada Department of Human Resources 960 F.2d 793 (9th Cir. 1992).
49. 15 USC #1012(b) and 15 USC #1013(b).

50. St. Paul Fire & Marine Insurance Co. v. Barry 438 US 531 (1978); Union Labor Life Insurance Co. v. Pireno 458 US 119 (1982); Group Life and Health Insurance Co. v. Royal Drug Co. 440 US 205 (1979); Ocean State Physicians Health Plan Inc. v. Blue Cross and Blue Shield of Rhode Island 883 F.2d 1101 (1st Cir. 1989).
51. 15 USC ## 34-36. Palm Spring Medical Clinic Inc. Desert Hospital 628 F. Supp. 454 (CD Cal. 1986); Tarabishi v. McAlester Regional Hospital 951 F.2d 1558 (10th Cir. 1991); See, however, R. Earnest Cohn DC v. Bond 953 F.2d 154 (4th Cir. 1991).
52. Summit Health Ltd. v. Pinhas 111 S Ct 1842 (1991). See also Fuentes v. South Hills Cardiology 946 F.2d 196 (3rd Cir. 1991).
53. Goldfarb v. Virginia State Bar Association 421 US 773 (1975).
54. See e.g. Standard Oil Co. v. US, 221 US 1, at 52 (1911) where the Court attributed a "deterioration of quality [to] monopolistic control of production and sale", and Northern Pacific Railway v. US 356 US 1 at 4 (1958) where the Court stated that competition assured the "... highest quality and the greatest material progress".
55. Goldfarb v. Virginia State Bar Association, at 788.
56. National Society of Professional Engineers v. US 435 US 679 (1978).
57. At p. 695-6.
58. Arizona v. Maricopa County Medical Society 457 US 332, at 345-48 (1981).
59. Jefferson Parish Hospital District No. 2 v. Hyde 446 US 2 (1984).
60. FTC. v. Indiana Federation of Dentists 476 US 447 (1986).
61. Indiana Federation of Dentists v. FTC 745 F.2d 1124 (7th Cir. 1984).
62. FTC v. Indiana Federation of Dentists, at 463.

Restatements and Conclusions

Providers, scholars, and policy-makers have during the past two decades concentrated on three major themes in medical care: cost, quality, and access. These issues have at times been discussed separately as if they could be isolated and conceptually compartmentalized. It is more likely, however, that these issues need to be analyzed in conjunction with each other, however complex the discussion then becomes. Cost, quality, and access in the health-care field are interwoven notions that should be examined simultaneously, even if it is not always easy or even possible. Diverging points of view introduced by different parties to the process complicate matters further. Providers, regulators, third-party payers, hospital administrators, and patient groups or their organized representatives, often take different, at times conflicting, approaches to the same problem depending upon their vested interest and political predisposition. In fact, these groups have often perceived these concepts differently, particularly quality, with access meaning different things to different people. Furthermore, each of these agents have displayed changing although normally predictable attitudes over the years.

We noted that healthcare quality also means different things to different people, but in general it seems to have meant to most people patient satisfaction, adherence to correct process, desirable outcome, all attained with significant efficiency - however any one or all of these terms are defined. Although the presence of this set of elements to quality is required, the individual elements can be quite independent from each other. Adherence to correct process was found not necessarily to result in desirable outcomes for every patient, at all stages of a disease, and at all times. Thus, care quality with these elements may be viewed as a macro concept applicable to a patient population as a whole in a general sense, taking on a different meaning or a different composition of elements in a micro context, that is, in relation to individual patients, specific ailments and time periods.

Whatever the definition, measurement and interpretation of healthcare quality and in whatever contexts, society requires it be sustained. At least in theory, somehow it must be enforced and policed. Here too, there is a divergence of enforcement approaches and philosophies. Historically, providers were expected to do their own policing through associations, speciality colleges, and other forms of member-based organizations, by the enforcement of various self-imposed ethical standards that normally placed the patient's interest and welfare in the forefront. Typically, however, the quality of healthcare given was likely to be more a function of the physician's own ethical standards than those imposed upon him or her from the outside. Hospitals implemented quality assurance programs through specialized groups, self-evaluation conferences, credentialing committees. Outside regulators aim at maintaining system-wide standards, although some of these, e.g. JCAHO, is the product of provider self-regulation. With the emergence of the federal government as a third-party payer, several regulatory programs were set in motion. These included the PSROs and later the PROs.

Notwithstanding these and other healthcare policing tools, tort law plays a role in healthcare quality policing. Issues pertaining to medical malpractice have been extensively discussed in the volume. It is by no means clear that the courts are in the position to set adequate medical practice standards, in spite of the usual array of medical expert witnesses on both sides of a litigation, or that the outcome of the litigation, whether by way of settlement, judgment, or verdict, can in fact be seen as a yardstick for measuring the extent to which any quality standards have been violated. Perhaps the best that can be said for the role of tort law in healthcare enforcement is that it may act as a source of fear, apprehension, and at times even prevention of gross negligence on the medical practice scene. But to the extent that it provokes "preventive medicine", however that may be distinguished from prudent medicine, it also interferes with efficiency and cost containment.

Who is or should be responsible for the quality of healthcare delivery in this convoluted, ever changing, and evolving environment? Who is or should be accountable for the infringement of quality standards? Traditionally, society looked to the physicians who also looked to themselves. However, economic, social, and political forces of the past two decades redirected at least part of the attention to patients, third-party payers, and governments. Until recent years, insurance coverage was virtually unlimited and insurance companies paid retrospectively almost any claim that was presented to them. Providers set their own fee, and charged for each and every service component performed. Physicians who charged a higher fee, or performed more services or more service components earned a higher income. Insurance companies rarely exercised their prerogative to reject a claim. Patients had no incentive to care about the cost of care because they paid very little or nothing out of their own pockets, and, because of the insurers' liberal payment policies, nor did physicians. If insurance company costs increased, those increases were simply passed on to business, and the latter at that time was much less healthcare costs sensitive than it became in recent years. A system of cost-shifting between those that paid and those that did not or could not allowed the care for the latter. New medical technology was developed and utilized, at a furious rate. Insurance companies and other third-party payers paid for them without much reservation and without any scrutiny as to their efficiency or need in the diagnostic or care process. Physicians had the economic power to delineate desirable care quality without much outside interference. Whatever care elements the physicians deemed as necessary for the patients, it would have been considered bad medicine not provide them, and for the carriers not pay for them. The ethics of medical practice of the time was consistent with this free-spending environment. The profession held physicians responsible for their patients' care. Patients were assumed to be passive participants in the care process to the extent that the AMA code of ethics, and even the Hippocratic Oath, empowered physicians to make all decisions for the patients, and to even withhold diagnostic and prognostic information except when patient input was absolutely needed for the treatment. Importantly, the cost of care was considered irrelevant to treatment decisions. It may have even been outright unethical to consider costs as a constraining factor in best treatment decisions, to reduce third-party payer's outlays, or to take into consideration political or social concerns for healthcare costs when planning or implementing such treatments.

The medicine of twenty or so years ago, at that time almost a sacred endeavor, saw money as no object or concern. However, consequent economic problems emerged at least in two dimensions: (a) national healthcare expenditures in the US have reached unprecedented highs at about one trillion dollars, around 14% of GDP, (b) the annual rate of growth in this expenditure has been increasing, until 1995 when the proliferation of managed care organizations appear to have had a small dampening impact. The latter slowdown in healthcare costs, however, could possibly be not only temporary but also nominal, for it may have been achieved at the expense of lower quality in some or most segments of the healthcare sector. The social benefits of slowed healthcare cost escalation may have been offset by increased social costs in terms of lower quality, and no one to my knowledge studied the net effect of this trade-off. This is not meant even to imply that this trade-off was or is in fact necessary, or that only the rate of cost escalation and quality were the only relevant variables in this trade-off. At any rate, preoccupation with healthcare costs is not a recent phenomenon. Efforts by way of regulating healthcare prices, controlling the proliferation of healthcare technology, and promoting healthy living so as to reduce system reliance, have been in place for many years. However, these efforts were implemented largely through various forms of a cost-plus, or the so called retrospective, payment system which, as we noted a number of times in the volume, held virtually no one accountable for healthcare costs. It is only during the past few years that various mechanisms were put in place to contain healthcare costs, or the cost containment function of existing mechanisms were intensified. These mechanisms included increasingly aggressive managed care, various internal and external peer review procedures, and cost saving financial incentives for providers. Third-party payers now negotiate reduced fee schedules, scrutinize care before it is given as to the care item's necessity and whether or not it is within the patient's contract. They often directly control physician decisions as to care as well as prescriptions, in addition to their indirect control of affiliated physicians by way of a system of financial incentives. Thus, an HMO affiliated doctor may find at the end of the year that his or her income is drastically affected by the number of hospitalizations he authorized, the number of tests she ordered, or the number of visits per patients the doctor entertained. If a treatment or diagnostic test is not ordered by the physician fearing that it will negatively impact on his or her financial or professional status, payers will not cover it, and hospitals will not perform it for they do not want to absorb the costs. The end result will likely be that, if the patient still wants it, the total cost, or a significant portion of it, will have to be absorbed by the patient. Thus, a certain segment of medical care gets rationed according to the financial means of the patient. The extent of the social injustice of this predicament is a function of the proportion of the patient-paid care that would be deemed as necessary in a professionally implemented fee-for-service payment regime, and of the extent to which patient-covered care generates a psychological benefit by way of peace of mind for the patient, benefit that is not available to those who cannot self-pay for it nor are they authorized to receive it.

An important underlying condition for the emergence of this predicament rests with the reduction or disappearance of bifurcation of economic resources, namely between control and ownership. In the past, physicians controlled healthcare resources almost literally with the stroke of a pen. They were their patients' agents. They ordered tests, diagnosed, ordered treatments, prescribed medications, and the third-party payer disbursed. No questions were asked. Care of quality was seen to depend on, and determined by, almost entirely the volume of tests, technology applied, and treatments ordered and implemented. More had to be better. The owners of healthcare resources, the hospitals, investors, insurance companies, other businesses, clinics and governments, asserted virtually no control over the medical care process of the physicians. All that has changed. Medical resource owners have also become controllers, in fact, were forced to become controllers by pressures from newly organized healthcare purchasing groups and by the proliferation of medical malpractice claims upon their healthcare resources. The characteristics of the consumer, the patient, have also changed. While in the past they were obedient and trusting of their physicians, they have now become demanding and suspicious, even litigious. Yet, somewhat paradoxically and in spite of these problems, and perhaps because a large proportion of the patient population is still insulated from the financial consequences of the care, patients still expect their physicians to be their exclusive, relentless and unselfish representatives of their interests. Many physicians still succeed in this difficult role. Rightfully so. Although many, if not most, patients are insulated from a large portion of the direct cost of their care, the patient population as a whole pays for the entire healthcare system. They do so through co-payments for the care, payment of their insurance premiums within and outside their employment environment, paying for the business' share of healthcare costs through higher product prices, and through taxes they pay for the government's entire contribution and role in the healthcare system. The healthcare system, all of its participants, patients, providers, businesses, governments, and other payers have become functionally, politically, socially, ethically, and, perhaps most importantly, economically interwoven into a network of competing yet interdependent entities, each seeking to protect or enhance their self-interests. Their perception or understanding of healthcare quality often differs with their vested interests. So does the manner whereby they attempt to serve the cause of healthcare quality as well as the method whereby they attempt to control healthcare costs.

HMOs and other managed care organizations have long been seen as bastions of healthcare cost control. Yet, notwithstanding the various means of financial control imposed on their affiliated providers, no such adequate financial constraints appears to be in place within their own organizations. Managed care entities should be viewed as at least quasi *public utilities* in many dimensions of their operation. Managed care executive remuneration and other elements of their operational costs and expenses should be scrutinized in a manner somewhat similar to the control that state public utility commissions impose upon their public utilities. Society with its healthcare system may not benefit any more from the very high, perhaps excessive, income levels of some managed care executives than it does from controlling provider incomes by various means in order to contain healthcare costs. There does not seem to be any notable evidence to the effect that healthcare quality varies proportionately or even directly with managed care executive remuneration. The old adage that high even exorbitant top executive income is at times returned to society by way of commensurately higher marginal productivity of the executives involved has at times been proven to be untrue in non-healthcare markets, and most likely had not had the time to be tested in healthcare markets. Yet, while many unanswered questions were raised by this volume, indeed, a purpose of the volume has been to draw attention to as many relevant issues related to the economics of healthcare quality as possible within its limited scope, one answer appears to have emerged. The era of dramatically spreading managed care environment is upon us. Just as importantly, it is accompanied by a rapidly increasing proportion of the population that will be older and in need of quality healthcare at a reasonable cost, however healthcare quality may be defined or measured. Thus, the social and economic justifications appear to be present for viewing managed care entities as a form of public utility. Issues related to the regulation of managed care costs, internal expenses, pricing, the anatomy of their providers' payment or reimbursement, and the quality of their services appear to have become prime targets for serious political and economic consideration.

Index